D0104102

Health Literacy in Nursing

Terri Ann Parnell, MA, DNP, RN, is principal and founder of Health Literacy Partners, LLC, a corporation that specializes in providing a tapestry of solutions to promote health equity by enhancing effective communication, person-centered care, and the patient experience. She is also assistant professor of population health at the Hofstra North Shore–LIJ School of Medicine, Hempstead, New York.

Prior to launching Health Literacy Partners, Dr. Parnell was the vice president for health literacy and patient education for the North Shore–LIJ Health System. In this role she was responsible for the health literacy strategic plan and the development, coordination, and implementation of all health literacy and patient education initiatives. She provided health literacy leadership and consultation for all departments and facilities across the North Shore–LIJ Health System, and was responsible for integrating concepts of health literacy, cultural awareness, and patient-centered care into core activities of the organization.

Dr. Parnell is a graduate of St. Vincent's Hospital School of Nursing (New York, New York) and earned her BSN from Adelphi University (Garden City, New York), a master's degree in health care administration from Hofstra University (Hempstead, New York), and her doctor of nursing practice degree from Case Western Reserve University (Cleveland, Ohio). Her graduate thesis researched health literacy knowledge and experience in senior-level baccalaureate nursing students.

With over 30 years' experience, including roles and responsibilities in patient education, health care administration, and nursing leadership, Dr. Parnell is well known for innovation in the area of health literacy. She has also received numerous nursing awards for excellence in research, patient and family education, and community service.

Dr. Parnell has served as a committee member on the American Nurses Association Care Coordination Quality Measures Panel and on the Institute of Medicine Roundtable on Health Literacy. She is coauthor of *Heart Smart for Black Women and Latinas: A Five-Week Program for Living a Heart-Healthy Lifestyle* (2008). Dr. Parnell is a frequent presenter locally, nationally, and internationally, and has published in the areas of women and heart disease, patient education, and health literacy.

Health Literacy in Nursing
Providing Person-Centered Care

Terri Ann Parnell, MA, DNP, RN

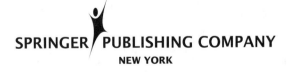

SPRINGER PUBLISHING COMPANY
NEW YORK

Copyright © 2015 Springer Publishing Company, LLC

All rights reserved.

No part of this publication may be reproduced, stored in a retrieval system, or transmitted in any form or by any means, electronic, mechanical, photocopying, recording, or otherwise, without the prior permission of Springer Publishing Company, LLC, or authorization through payment of the appropriate fees to the Copyright Clearance Center, Inc., 222 Rosewood Drive, Danvers, MA 01923, 978-750-8400, fax 978-646-8600, info@copyright.com or on the Web at www.copyright.com.

Springer Publishing Company, LLC
11 West 42nd Street
New York, NY 10036
www.springerpub.com

Acquisitions Editor: Margaret Zuccarini
Composition: diacriTech

ISBN: 978-0-8261-6172-7
e-book ISBN: 978-0-8261-6173-4

14 15 16 / 5 4 3 2 1

The author and the publisher of this Work have made every effort to use sources believed to be reliable to provide information that is accurate and compatible with the standards generally accepted at the time of publication. The author and publisher shall not be liable for any special, consequential, or exemplary damages resulting, in whole or in part, from the readers' use of, or reliance on, the information contained in this book. The publisher has no responsibility for the persistence or accuracy of URLs for external or third-party Internet websites referred to in this publication and does not guarantee that any content on such websites is, or will remain, accurate or appropriate.

Library of Congress Cataloging-in-Publication Data

Health literacy in nursing : providing person-centered care / [edited by] Terri Ann Parnell.
    p. ; cm.
Includes bibliographical references.
ISBN 978-0-8261-6172-7 — ISBN 978-0-8261-6173-4 (e-book)
I. Parnell, Terri Ann, editor.
[DNLM: 1. Health Literacy. 2. Nursing Care—methods. 3. Communication. 4. Patient Education as Topic. 5. Patient-Centered Care. WY 100.1]
    RA427
    362.1—dc23

                            2014010967

Special discounts on bulk quantities of our books are available to corporations, professional associations, pharmaceutical companies, health care organizations, and other qualifying groups. If you are interested in a custom book, including chapters from more than one of our titles, we can provide that service as well.

For details, please contact:
Special Sales Department
Springer Publishing Company, LLC
11 West 42nd Street, 15th Floor
New York, NY 10036-8002
Phone: 877-687-7476 or 212-431-4370
Fax: 212-941-7842
E-mail: sales@springerpub.com

Printed in the United States of America by McNaughton & Gunn.

I dedicate this book to Aubrey and Max.
I am so proud that they are part of the future generation
of nursing professionals.

Contents

Contributors

Gloria M. Collura, MS, RNC-NIC
Director of Patient Care Services
Pediatric Perioperative Service
Cohen Children's Medical Center
North Shore–LIJ Health System
New Hyde Park, New York

Fallon Edwards, MPH
Project Manager, Health Literacy and Patient Education
Office of Diversity, Inclusion and Health Literacy
North Shore–LIJ Health System
Lake Success, New York

Hallie Kassan, MS
Director
Office of the Human Research Protection Program
North Shore–LIJ Health System
New Hyde Park, New York

Elizabeth C. McCulloch, MS, PhD(c)
Director, Language Access Services and Performance Improvement
Office of Diversity, Inclusion and Health Literacy
North Shore–LIJ Health System
Lake Success, New York

Jennifer H. Mieres, MD, FACC, FASNC, FAHA
Senior Vice President
Office of Community and Public Health
Chief Diversity and Inclusion Officer
Medical Director, Center for Learning and Innovation
North Shore–LIJ Health System
Great Neck, New York
Professor of Cardiology and Population Health
Hofstra North Shore–LIJ School of Medicine
Hempstead, New York

Suzanne Monteleone, MS, RNC-NIC
Director of Nursing Education and Professional Development
Cohen Children's Medical Center
North Shore–LIJ Health System
New Hyde Park, New York

Terri Ann Parnell, MA, DNP, RN
Principal and Founder
Health Literacy Partners, LLC
Garden City, New York
Assistant Professor of Population Health
Hofstra North Shore–LIJ School of Medicine
Hempstead, New York

Joanne Turnier, MS, RN, ACNS-BC, CNRN, CT
Director of Health Literacy and Patient Education
Office of Diversity, Inclusion and Health Literacy
North Shore–LIJ Health System
Lake Success, New York

Foreword

The worlds of science and health are moving at unprecedented speed. If we are not careful, the population we serve, and even our colleagues, will be in danger of being left behind as the complexity and tsunami of emerging science continue to evolve. The timely translation of complex, health-related scientific information to the end user is essential to the health of individuals, communities, and the nation.

Health literacy, the ability to effectively translate this evolving content to the end user to effect understanding and sustainable behavioral change, is inextricably tied to cultural competence, for we must also understand the context, culture, and environment of the people we have the privilege to serve. Although it has been almost 14 years since health literacy was first discussed as a necessary component of health promotion, the actual effective use of health literacy is still in its infancy.

Health literacy should be embedded in all public health endeavors as well as multidisciplinary health professional education. For several years the Institute of Medicine has conducted a roundtable on health literacy to bring together the foremost thought leaders in health literacy in order to define best practices and raise awareness of this concept that is essential to the public's health.

In her textbook, Dr. Parnell has captured the essence of health literacy and cultural competence, not only for nurses, but also applicable to all care providers and community workers. As a former registered nurse I recognize the immense and unique role that my nursing colleagues play in the practice and teaching of health literacy and cultural competence. Long before the concepts of health literacy and cultural competence were formulated, nursing was on the forefront of effective health communication. Today, once again, with new knowledge and technology, nursing leads the way in effecting sustainable health-related behavioral change and cultural competence.

Most of the disease and economic burdens on us are because of poor lifestyle choices, which are amenable to behavioral change if we embrace health literacy and cultural competence in all our endeavors. *Health Literacy in Nursing: Providing Person-Centered Care* provides us with a road map to enhance our success through health literacy and cultural competence. This is a must read for all health professionals.

Richard H. Carmona, MD, MPH, FACS
17th Surgeon General of the United States (2002–2006)
Distinguished Professor, University of Arizona, Tucson, Arizona

Preface

Health Literacy in Nursing: Providing Person-Centered Care is, first and foremost, written as a guide for all those in the nursing profession, who are new graduate nurses or experienced nurses. As stated by Dr. Richard H. Carmona, 17th Surgeon General of the United States (2002–2006), "Health literacy is the currency for success in everything we do in health, wellness, and prevention." It is a crosscutting priority for all nurses, whether practicing in ambulatory or inpatient care, acute or chronic care, specialty care, adult or pediatric care, nursing research, or community and transitional care. Health literacy is vital to prevention, wellness, and illness, and must be woven throughout the fabric of all that we do in nursing.

This book is written to provide a general overview of health literacy, as it is difficult to incorporate a comprehensive illustration of every type of health literacy encounter. It is divided into four parts with specific chapters within each part for quick and easy reference.

Part I, "Health Literacy: The Magnitude of the Issue," provides an overall baseline knowledge of health literacy. Chapter 1 illustrates the history of health literacy and health literacy definitions, as well as conceptual and theoretical models. Chapter 2 defines low or limited health literacy and the implications of low health literacy to the professionals providing health care and to the individuals receiving the care. Chapter 3 discusses the changing demographics and the delivery of person-centered care in a diverse environment. Chapter 4 touches on health literacy and its impact on accessing care and navigating throughout a complex health care delivery system. Chapter 5, the last chapter in Part I, reviews the major health literacy efforts of the federal government, scientists, health researchers, health policy experts, and health professionals.

Part II focuses on the role of oral communication. Chapter 6 discusses effective oral communication and defines plain language, also known as "living room language." Chapter 7 incorporates the role and importance of culture, language, and communication access services needed to provide quality, safe person-centered care. Chapter 8 closes Part II with a focus on nursing strategies to enhance effective communication and understanding. It provides strategies that nurses can incorporate into their daily care that can have a vital impact upon effective communication.

Part III focuses on written health communication and begins with Chapter 9, the development of written content for health information and for educational materials. Chapter 10 discusses content design and layout of written health information and patient education. How written information is presented can have a tremendous impact on readability and understandability.

Health Literacy in Nursing: Providing Person-Centered Care concludes with Part IV, which helps to prepare nurses who care for unique populations. The chapters incorporated in "Health Literacy and Unique Populations" are written by select authors who bring their expertise when caring for specific patient populations. Chapter 11 presents health literacy implications when caring for persons in palliative care and making difficult end-of-life decisions. The changing landscape of death and dying, the significant changes in the way Americans die, and how to integrate health literacy strategies into palliative care discussions are addressed.

Chapter 12 identifies the uniqueness of caring for young children and how the parents' or caregivers' health literacy level impacts the care, decisions, and treatment for young children and adolescents. The uniqueness of health literacy and children's health and ways to enhance both child and parent health literacy are illustrated. Chapter 13 focuses on the challenges and opportunities faced by nurses caring for patients with mental health disorders. This chapter reviews the implications of low health literacy and mental health disorders upon one's feeling of stigma and shame, knowledge about illness and treatment, and attitudes, recognition, and task shifting. Chapter 14 portrays the "graying of America" and the demographic trends that are occurring as the U.S. population ages. Research regarding health literacy and age-related challenges, such as sensory and cognitive changes, are discussed. Lastly, Chapter 15 presents the ethical principles of human research subjects, how to ensure that research participants with low health literacy are protected, and how to uphold the principles of the Belmont

Report. The contributions each of these select authors have made to this book deserve special thanks and recognition.

Health literacy represents the weaving of life experiences and behaviors between an individual and the professionals providing health care—be it prevention, wellness, or sick care. It is my hope that the reader who uses this book will find that the information enhances his or her awareness, knowledge, and understanding of health literacy and provides both nursing strategies and a platform to further discuss and research with colleagues.

—*Terri Ann Parnell*

Acknowledgments

I would first like to thank my husband and family for their ongoing support, encouragement, and love.

Special thanks and appreciation to each of my contributing chapter authors for their camaraderie and willingness to share their health literacy passion and subject matter expertise.

My sincere gratitude to Dr. Richard H. Carmona for his insightful Foreword.

I wish to thank Margaret Zuccarini and the entire team at Springer Publishing Company for the opportunity to create this textbook. It has been a pleasure to work with each of you.

From my earliest memories I wanted to be a nurse. I am not sure where the idea came from. I do know that I always wanted to work in a field that would help people. Although no one in my immediate family was in nursing, my grandmother, whom I adored, worked as an administrator in the admitting department of a hospital. My family and I often visited the hospital to see her and came to know the staff as our extended family.

It made perfect sense, therefore, for me to begin my professional career in the same hospital as a "new diploma nursing graduate." Young, but confident in my training, I was able to go right into the surgical intensive care unit. Traumas, bleeders, and suicide jumpers were among my first patients. It was truly intense, especially for a new nursing graduate.

Almost 35 years later, the memories are as fresh in my mind as if it were yesterday.

After a year I moved to a hospital in the suburbs. It would soon be time to settle down and have a family. When that time arrived, I was able to change my work schedule to adapt to some of the milestones in my personal life. My nursing career continued to grow and evolve. A bachelor's degree in nursing was followed by a master's degree in health care administration and ultimately a doctorate in nursing practice over a 25-year span.

Today when I am asked, "What do you do?" the answer is always the same. First and foremost, "I am a nurse." Only then do I continue to explain my actual role and responsibilities. My perspective would not be the same if I didn't have my foundation in nursing. Nurses look at things differently. Collectively we have a keen ability to multitask, shift directions in an instant, and still have the compassion and empathy for the person and family we are caring for. After all, they are the reason we are here.

I feel extremely blessed to get up each day and do something I truly love. Nursing has been very good to me. I only hope that I can continue to return the favor to the nursing profession.

This book could not have been possible without the foundational education and experiences from the patients, faculty, staff, employees, and community of St. Vincent's Hospital and St. Vincent's School of Nursing in New York City. Thank you and I miss you!

Health Literacy: The Magnitude
of the Issue

Health Literacy:
History, Definitions, and Models

Terri Ann Parnell

As the field of health literacy expands in scope and breadth, the term health literacy continues to have a plethora of meanings depending on whom you are speaking to and the context of reference. It can have an extremely broad reference, such as when referring to the health literacy environment of a health care organization or health care system. Health literacy can also have a very specific reference, such as when referring to an individual's health literacy skills when visiting a physician's office for the first time or accessing an emergency department for acute chest pain. Historically, many felt health literacy skills were dependent purely upon individual skills and abilities while others expressed that they were dependent upon the skills or abilities of the "system" or health care organization. Fortunately, there has been a recent shift toward the understanding that health literacy is about the relationship between the skills of persons receiving care or treatment and the professionals or systems that are providing the care and treatment. An individual's health literacy skills are dynamic and change over time depending on the context, changes in individual skills and experiences, or changes in the health care system. Health literacy continues to be an evolving concept that has more recently been viewed as a crosscutting priority in the delivery of safe, quality health care.

3

In 1992, the National Adult Literacy Survey was completed in the United States. It measured the ability of adults to use written information for everyday tasks and focused on reading, writing, and arithmetic. It demonstrated that nearly half of American adults are at a disadvantage when faced with the literacy demands encountered in everyday life.

In 2003, the U.S. Department of Education, National Center for Education Statistics completed the National Assessment of Adult Literacy (NAAL; Kutner, Greenberg, Jin, & Paulson, 2006). This was conducted with the goal of measuring the status of English adult literacy in the United States and for the first time included a specific section to measure health literacy. The health literacy section focused on the ability to read, understand, and apply health-related information in English (White, 2008) and focused on health tasks that were grouped into clinical, preventive, and navigation of the health system categories. As reported in the NAAL, many adults have difficulty functioning in the health care system due to a lack of health literacy skills. And according to the American Medical Association (AMA) report (Weiss, 2007) *Health Literacy and Patient Safety: Help Patients Understand,* "poor health literacy is a stronger predictor of a person's health status than age, income, employment status, education level and race." Additional research has shown that even well-educated persons of all ages, races, and socioeconomic levels can experience low health literacy as they are expected to take on more responsibility for prevention and self-management of chronic illness.

In 2013, the National Center for Education Statistics reported results from the most recent adult literacy assessment, the Program for the International Assessment of Adult Competencies (PIAAC). Twenty-four countries from around the world participated in the PIAAC. In the United States, the study was completed in 2011 to 2012 with a nationally representative sample of 5,000 adults between the ages of 16 and 65. The goal of the study was to assess and compare the basic skills and range of competencies of adults from around the world (Goodman, Finnegan, Mohadjer, Krenzke, & Hogan, 2013, p. 1). The PIAAC defined four core competency domains of adult cognitive skills including literacy, reading components, numeracy, and problem solving in technology-rich environments. PIAAC defined the domains as below:

- Literacy as "understanding, evaluating, using and engaging in written text to participate in society, achieve one's goals and to develop one's knowledge and potential."

- Reading components focused the assessment on elements of reading that were comparable across the scope of languages in all participating countries including vocabulary, sentence comprehension, and basic passage comprehension.

- Numeracy as "the ability to access, use, interpret, and communicate mathematical information and ideas, to engage in and manage mathematical demands of a range of situations in adult life."
- Problem solving in technology-rich environments as "using digital technology, communication tools, and networks to acquire and evaluate information, communicate with others, and perform practical tasks" (Organisation for Economic Co-operation and Development, 2012)

The United States assessed all four domains; however, only the literacy and numeracy domains were required to be assessed by all participating countries. Tasks within each domain were designed from culturally appropriate real-life experiences in an effort to reflect how groups of adults perform in their daily activities. PIAAC results are reported on a scale of 0 to 500 and as percentages of adults that met established proficiency levels. Although the complex relationships between the data variables have yet to be fully explored, the purpose of the First Look report is intended to introduce the data, initially through figures, tables, and selected findings (Goodman et al., 2013, p. 1). Unfortunately, there was no formal health literacy component as there was in the 2003 NAAL. Selected findings related to adults ages 16 to 65 in the United States are reported as follows (PIAAC, 2012):

- Literacy domain:
  - The United States was below the international average with a score of 270. Average scores in 12 countries were significantly higher, average scores in five countries were significantly lower, and in five countries there was no significant difference.

- Numeracy domain:
  - The United States scored third to last in numeracy skills with an average score of 253. The only countries scoring below the United States were Italy and Spain.

- Problem-solving in technology-rich environments domain:
  - The United States was below the PIAAC international average with an average score of 277. Ireland scored the same and the only remaining country that scored lower was Poland with an average score of 275.

The PIACC is a very complex assessment that builds upon previous international assessment data and experience. The PIAAC assessment conducted in the United States was done only in English, although the background items were in both English and Spanish.

The First Look report provides important results that need further analysis. However, initial data continue to provide important results that emphasize the ongoing national efforts necessary to enhance the literacy and numeracy skills of U.S. adults. Although there was not a specific health literacy domain, low literacy and numeracy skills have a direct relationship upon an individual's health literacy skills. Low health literacy remains a crosscutting priority that is a threat to the health of all Americans and health care organizations.

Definitions of Health Literacy

The term health literacy was first used in 1974 to describe how health information impacts the educational system, the health care system, and mass communication and was used as a goal to be established for grades K through 12 (AMA, 2005, p. 4). The concept of health literacy was not introduced into health care literature until the 1990s and the emphasis on self-management of health and disease in the early 2000s has placed more of a focus on an individual's health literacy skills (Cutilli & Bennett, 2009). Health literacy as a concept has progressed from describing and defining the literacy skills of the adult population to the understanding that adequate, if not advanced, literacy skills are necessary to access, navigate, and understand the health care system of today.

Early definitions of health literacy focused on the ability of an individual to apply basic reading and numeracy skills to a health care concept, as in the degree to which individuals have the capacity to obtain, process, and understand basic health information and services needed to make appropriate health decisions (Institute of Medicine [IOM], 2004; Ratzan & Parker, 2000). Minor changes were suggested to this definition after consultation with an expert panel and review of other definitions found in the literature. The modified definition substituted "the capacity to" with "can" in an effort to emphasize the measurement of ability and separate health literacy from intelligence. It also added "communicate about" to emphasize the importance of oral communication skills. The term "basic" was suggested being removed, as each health literacy experience requires differing types of information and the term "health services" was eliminated. The word "informed" was suggested as a substitute for "appropriate," as cultural preferences may influence interactions with the health care system and professionals (Berkman, Davis, & McCormack, 2010). Based on the stated suggestions, this revised definition of health literacy reads as "the degree to which individuals can obtain, process, understand, and communicate about health-related information needed to make informed health decisions."

The World Health Organization (WHO) expands the definition to include personal action or use of information and states that health literacy represents the cognitive and social skills that determine the motivation and ability of individuals to gain access to, understand, and use information in ways that promote and maintain good health (WHO, 1998, p. 10). The AMA's Ad Hoc Committee on Health Literacy (1999) describes health literacy as "the constellation of skills, including the ability to perform basic reading and numerical tasks required to function in the health care environment," including the ability to read and comprehend prescription bottles.

Ratzan (2001) defines health literacy as a framework for health promotion activities and a link between knowledge and practice.

Health literacy has also been defined with a focus on health promotion, such as "the personal, cognitive, and social skills which determine the ability of individuals to gain access and understand, and use information to promote and maintain good health" by Nutbeam (2000). Another definition defines health literacy as an evolving lifetime process that includes the attributes of capacity, comprehension, and communication (Mancuso, 2008).

Other experts express health literacy as being a dynamic state and define health literacy as a "wide range of skills that people develop to seek out, comprehend, evaluate and use health information and concepts to make informed choices, reduce risks and increase quality of life." This definition implies that individuals' health literacy skills can change depending on various health experiences (Zarcadoolas, Pleasant, & Greer, 2005).

Health literacy affects all health care efforts and is based on the interaction of a person's skills with health contexts, health care and education systems, and broad social and cultural factors at home, work, and in the community (IOM, 2011a).

Still others state that definitions of health literacy should incorporate the role of language and cultural and social constructs. It is "a tapestry of skills combining basic literacy, math skills, and a belief in the basic tenets of the treatment modality" (McCabe, 2006). To further expand on the concept of a "tapestry of skills," health literacy requires a true partnership and cannot be simply looked upon as a measurement of an individual's literacy skills. Health literacy is "dependent upon individual and system factors, which also include the communication skills, knowledge, and culture of both the professional and lay person, the context as well as the demands of the health care and public health system" (Berkman et al., 2010). This concept of health literacy removes the sole responsibility from the layperson and shares it with the clinicians and health care system.

After a systematic review of the literature regarding definitions of health literacy, Sorensen et al. (2012) deviated from the basic concept that health literacy is a skill set. "Health literacy is linked to literacy and entails people's knowledge, motivation, and competence to access, understand, appraise and apply health information in order to make judgments and take decisions in everyday life concerning health care, disease prevention, and health promotion to maintain or improve quality of life during the life-course" (Sorensen et al., 2012, p. 3).

The wide range of health literacy definitions (Table 1.1), the continued discussions on whether health literacy is an individual or system skill, if it is stagnant or dynamic, all contribute to the challenges of continued research, consistent measurement, and possible solutions to enhancing low health literacy. Health literacy must be at the forefront of all that we do in nursing and health care. Clinicians can begin by reflecting on any unconscious bias that may be present, and reassessing their communication skills. Avoiding the use of medical jargon, respectfully using question-and-answer format and incorporating the use of teach-back for ascertaining understanding can assist in enhancing an individual's health literacy skills. Clinicians can also assess opportunities that could enhance ease of navigation when accessing health care services.

Table 1.1 Definitions of Health Literacy

World Health Organization	1998	"Cognitive and social skills which determine the motivation and ability of individuals to gain access to, understand, and use information in ways that promote and maintain good health."
American Medical Association	1999	"The constellation of skills, including the ability to perform basic reading and numerical tasks required to function in the health care environment."
Nutbeam	2000	"The personal, cognitive, and social skills which determine the ability of individuals to gain access and understand, and use information to promote and maintain good health."
Institute of Medicine	2004	"The degree to which individuals have the capacity to obtain, process, and understand basic health information and services needed to make appropriate health decisions."
Zarcadoolas, Pleasant, & Greer	2005	"A wide range of skills that people develop to seek out, comprehend, evaluate and use health information and concepts to make informed choices, reduce risks and increase quality of life."

(continued)

Table 1.1 Definitions of Health Literacy (*continued*)

McCabe	2006	"A tapestry of skills combining basic literacy, math skills, and a belief in the basic tenets of the treatment modality."
Mancuso	2008	"An evolving lifetime process that includes the attributes of capacity, comprehension and communication."
Freedman et al.	2009	"The degree to which individuals and groups can obtain, process, understand, evaluate, and act upon information needed to make public health decisions that benefit the community."
Berkman, Davis, & McCormack	2010	"Dependent upon individual and system factors, which also include the communication skills, knowledge, and culture of both the professional and lay person, the context as well as the demands of the health care and public health system."
Patient Protection and Affordable Care Act of 2010	2010	"The degree to which an individual has the capacity to obtain, communicate, process, and understand basic health information and services to make appropriate health decisions."
Sorensen et al.	2012	"Health literacy is linked to literacy and entails people's knowledge, motivation, and competence to access, understand, appraise and apply health information in order to make judgements and take decisions in everyday life concerning healthcare, disease prevention, and health promotion to maintain or improve quality of life during the life-course."

Others feel that a brand new type of health literacy is needed to incorporate the influences of globalization and poverty and state that the current variety of definitions pose many limitations (Freedman et al., 2009).

Public health literacy is defined as "the degree to which individuals and groups can obtain, process, understand, evaluate, and act upon information needed to make public health decisions that benefit the community" (Freedman et al., 2009, p. 448).

The Patient Protection and Affordable Care Act of 2010 (ACA) defines health literacy as the degree to which an individual has the capacity to obtain, communicate, process, and understand basic health information and services to make appropriate health decisions (Centers for Disease Control and Prevention [CDC], 2010). This definition is similar to the Healthy People definition with the addition of the term "communicate."

Healthy People 2010 and 2020 incorporated improving the health literacy of the population as a specific objective (U.S. Department of Health and Human Services [USDHHS], 2010). In the IOM report *Health Literacy: A Prescription to End Confusion* (2004), it is stated that "health literacy emerges when the expectations, preferences, and skills of those seeking information and services meet the expectations, preferences, and skills of those providing information and services." Health literacy is not an individual issue and this definition exemplifies the partnership that is necessary to truly provide person-centered care. It will take more than individual skills to change health behavior and ultimately address the health and prevention challenges we currently face and will continue to face in the future.

Magnitude of the Issue

When reflecting on patient- or health-related research, reading ability and literacy skills as they relate to comprehension were the initial focus reported in the literature in the 1980s and 1990s (Speros, 2005). Those in the field of health literacy owe a tremendous amount of appreciation for the early research done by Leonard and Cecilia Doak and Jane Root. Doak, Doak, and Root helped to demonstrate the gap that existed between health education materials and a person's lack of comprehension and this was shared in their publication *Teaching Patients with Low Literacy Skills* (Doak, Doak, & Root, 1996).

As a nurse, do you routinely think of your patients' reading ability when giving them their discharge summary? When handing your patient a clipboard with admission forms to complete, do you offer to help with filling it out? How do you really know that your preoperative instructions were understood by asking, "Do you have any questions?"

The NAAL, completed by the Department of Education in 2003, is the only national assessment tool to have a specific component to measure health literacy. Over 19,000 U.S. adults age 16 and older participated in the national and state-level assessments, most in their homes and some in prisons from the 50 states and the District of Columbia.

The NAAL assessed adults' prose, document, and quantitative literacy ability along with printed materials that are encountered on a daily basis when undergoing activities while at home, at work, or in the community (Figure 1.1).

An example of finding and using information from continuous text known as prose literacy is reading a brochure or instructional information. It requires the person to read text in a paragraph, to search and comprehend the content. Following preoperative or preprocedure instructions is an example of prose literacy. Document literacy incorporates the ability to read noncontinuous text such

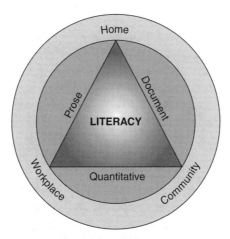

Figure 1.1 Framework for the 2003 National Assessment of Adult Literacy.
Source: White and McCloskey (forthcoming). *Framework for the 2003 National Assessment of Adult Literacy* (NCES 2005-531). U.S. Department of Education. Washington, DC: National Center for Education Statistics.

as forms, charts, or labels. In health care, document literacy is necessary for the completion of history forms on admission or comprehension of specific charts. Quantitative literacy incorporates the computation of numbers in the content being read. An example of quantitative literacy specific to health care is medication dosing or reading about the percentage of risk related to a specific procedure.

All health-related tasks in the NAAL fit into the prose, document, and quantitative scales but were related only to health content. The health literacy section specifically assessed the ability of adults to use their literacy skills when trying to understand health-related information in the clinical, prevention, and navigation areas with the majority of items being preventive and navigation as they are more applicable to the majority of the population.

The NAAL categorized health literacy into four separate categories including below basic, basic, intermediate, and proficient, and reported the following overall results (Figure 1.2).

It demonstrated that the majority of adults exhibited intermediate health literacy; however, more than one third or 36% of the adult population had basic or below basic health literacy (retrieved from nces.ed.gov/naal/health_results.asp, cited as Kutner et al., 2006). The results of the NAAL illustrated that individuals who have the most difficulty understanding health information are 65 years of age or older, Black or Hispanic, male, live at or below the poverty level, spoke another language before their formal education, are either uninsured or have

Overall

Total Population: Number and Percentage of Adults in Each Health Literacy Level: 2003

- A majority of adults had *Intermediate* heath literacy.
- Over 75 million adults combined had *Basic* and *Below Basic* health literacy.

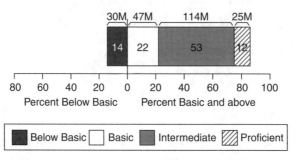

Figure 1.2 Overall NAAL results.

Medicaid or Medicare, and do not seek information from print or nonprint sources more often than persons with higher levels of health literacy (Kutner et al., 2006). This provides us with a baseline of literacy and health literacy skills of American adults and assists in identifying the populations in greatest need.

The nursing profession represents the largest group of the U.S. health care workforce and has close proximity to the patient (IOM, 2011b). As nurses we must provide information in a way that is understandable to all patients and therefore would benefit from incorporating a "universal approach" when providing health education. After all, the NAAL reported that only 12% of adults in the United States exhibit proficient health literacy skills, indicating that health literacy is indeed a crosscutting priority. Health literacy should be a critical concern for everyone involved in wellness, health promotion, disease prevention, and treatment and management of chronic illness. Nurses directly and profoundly affect the quality of care patients receive and can make a positive impact by addressing the critical role of health literacy (Murphy-Knoll, 2007).

Misconceptions and Unconscious Bias

What are the assumptions or misconceptions that we may unconsciously make when it comes to health literacy? There are many—some much more obvious than others. Let's take some time to go through and discuss them. This will allow us to pause and reflect on how we practice and what our expectations are for those we care for.

Misconception #1

Patients fully understand health information and instructions that were taught simply because they nod "yes" when asked or when they nod "no" when asked if they have any questions.

Ask your nursing colleagues if their patients always understand what they have explained? I am sure you will get overwhelming positive responses, such as "Yes, they understand" or "Do you think I would send my patients home if they didn't understand what to do!" The majority of nurses go into the field because they want to help others. They truly care about their patients and would never do anything intentional to cause harm. In fact, many nurses have responded to the above question with, "Yes, of course they understand. I even ask my patients if they have any questions and they nod 'no.' I make an effort to spend time with my patients and I teach all of my patients before they are discharged." What does that negative nod really mean? Perhaps it means, "I need to leave right now so that I can get home in time to pick up my daughter from school"; or maybe, "I don't want my nurse to think I am dumb," or even, "My nurse seems so busy, I don't want to take up any more time." Shame plays an important role when attempting to understand how low-literate patients interact with their health care providers in the health care setting (Parikh, Parker, Nurss, Baker, & Williams, 1996). Even well-educated, literate patients may feel shame and embarrassment and not want to admit they do not understand. In a study by Castro, Wilson, Wang, and Schillinger (2007), there was a reported mismatch between patients self-reported understanding and the clinicians overestimate of patient understanding when simply asking patients, "Do you understand?" Nurses and health care professionals often provide too much complex information that is not necessary for the patient and family to know. An affirmative response by the patient indicating understanding of the information taught may simply mean that the patient did not feel empowered to speak up. There may also be generational or cultural reasons why the patient nods in acknowledgment even when they do not understand. Most persons will not openly admit that they do not understand the information provided.

Misconception #2

Substituting plain language for medical jargon is insulting to well-educated persons.

Communication plays such a vital role in the delivery of safe and effective health care. Nurses often assume that when we are educating our patients that communication is occurring. Try for a moment to place yourself in your patient's place. You are an educated professional, maybe even with advanced degrees. How would you feel if you were asked to do something very unfamiliar for the first time, such as change the brakes on your car? Imagine if the process was explained to you once and then you were given "simple instructions" to follow as in the below excerpt.

Replacing your car brakes involves a series of simple steps, as follows:

i.   Allow all the components of the braking mechanism—the rotor, calipers and the pads to cool down completely.

ii. Clean all the moving parts with cleaner and remove the braking fluid from the master cylinder using a siphoning device.

iii. Loosen the lug nuts and then, with the help of a lifting jack, raise your vehicle and place a jack stand underneath to keep it locked in place. Now remove the lug nuts completely from the wheel to access the braking assembly.

iv. Loosen the bolts and take out the brake calipers. Use cleaning lube to clean it or if it looks damaged, replace it with a new set. (www .instructables.com)

The above instructions are written in terms unfamiliar to many of us who are not in the industry of automobile mechanics. Some would say that the excerpt uses "automobile-eze" or a language that is foreign to us. Would you be able to follow these "simple instructions?" I would venture to say that for many, probably not. I would consider myself an educated professional, yet I don't know what a rotor or caliper are or what they would even look like! Why, then, do we assume that our patients understand our medical language or jargon? Persons with low health literacy have difficulty understanding information related to health, just as you may have difficulty understanding information related to automobile mechanics. Using plain, everyday language is not insulting or "dumbing down" and is helpful to all consumers of health care.

Misconception #3

All persons with low health literacy skills are uneducated and cannot read or write.

When speaking to nurses and other health care professionals about health literacy and low health literacy it is often stated, "Yes, I understand about low health literacy, but it doesn't apply to my patients. You see, our patient demographic is primarily White, well-educated, and from a high socioeconomic group. We don't have to worry about low health literacy here." This is a common response. There is a general misconception when it comes to identifying persons with low health literacy in a more homogeneous, educated, affluent patient population.

A nationally known general surgeon was admitted to the hospital for open-heart surgery. He was scheduled for a triple bypass and as the nurse was preparing him for surgery I asked if she had the opportunity to teach him about what to expect before, during, and after the surgery. She stated, "He is a surgeon, I am sure he knows what to expect. I asked if he had any questions when I was admitting him and he shook his head and said 'no'." As nurses, we must not assume that our patients have certain skill sets based on a title or profession that implies many years of education. In this situation, although the general surgeon was an expert in his field, he may not have all the knowledge when it comes to another subspecialty. In fact, this would be a wonderful opportunity to individualize the teaching to his needs and foundational knowledge base.

Misconception #4

I will be able to tell if my patient cannot read the information provided. Anyway, my patient will tell me if he or she cannot read.

Persons who have some difficulty reading have often developed a keen ability to adapt and function throughout their life. There is the story of a gentleman in his mid-60s, who had just retired and was now afforded the opportunity to spend more time with his grandchildren. His two grandchildren would climb up into his lap and ask, "Pop-pop, can you read us a story?" He would struggle as he tried to read a storybook to his very young grandchildren and at times would even make excuses that he was busy. Finally, he got the courage to tell his wife of over 40 years that he had difficulty reading. He was so ashamed. As you might imagine she was extremely shocked. "What do you mean you can't read!? We have been together our entire life, you held down a great job, we own a home and put two children through college?" He embarrassingly said, "I can read a little, I was able to figure it out. I would buy the newspaper every day so the guys at work wouldn't find out. When we were getting our coffee in the morning I would ask about the game that was on the night before, I would say I fell asleep and missed the ending. Or I would listen to the radio to hear the current events. But now that I can't read to my grandchildren . . . it is too much of a burden to continue on this way."

He went to an adult literacy center in town and was tutored and was able to eventually read stories to his grandchildren. He went his entire life without anyone ever finding out. He would make up excuses like "I forgot my glasses, can I take this home with me to fill out?" or "My wife takes care of things like this." No one ever suspected. Research by Parikh et al. (1996) reported that two-thirds of 58 patients who admitted having reading difficulties had never told their spouse. One half never told their children. Nine of them had told no one. Many persons with low literacy are able to keep it very well hidden by bringing someone with them to appointments, making excuses, or even worse, by pretending to be able to read. A key phrase to remember is "you can't tell by looking." This is accurately demonstrated in the 2001 video by the AMA, "Low Health Literacy: You Can't Tell by Looking," as it showcases the interaction between real patients with physicians and office staff. Over and over we hear this phrase: "Of course my patient would tell me if she could not read what I gave her!" The reality is that there is a tremendous amount of shame and embarrassment associated with limited literacy and the majority of poor readers will not easily share this information. Common reasons for not signing or completing a basic history or demographic intake form are that the person "left his reading glasses at home" or "my spouse always fills this in for me, she has all the information so I will take it home and then bring it back." Sometimes the person may state that "you already have this information from my last visit; why do I need to complete this again" and even become angry and leave without being seen. Although we should not stereotype that all persons who behave in this manner or make these statements have low literacy skills, we should be cognizant that these reasons may actually be indicative of an individual who could benefit from respectful assistance in completing paperwork.

Misconception #5

The number of years of education is a good indicator of an individual's health literacy skills.

The number of years of completed education is just that—how many years of formal schooling the person completed. It is not necessarily an accurate indicator of the health literacy skills an individual may have. In fact, when it comes to reading, surveys have indicated that on average, people read several grade levels lower than the number of school years completed. A nurse with advanced education and over 25 years experience in trauma nursing is diagnosed with multiple sclerosis. She makes an appointment with a nationally known neurologist at the hospital where she is employed. The physician recognizes her as an employee of many years and makes an effort to go into a tremendous amount of detailed explanation about her test results. He is trying to be helpful and complete in his explanation, as she is a well-respected nurse. She is anxious and frightened; after all, she knows someone who was recently diagnosed with MS and within 18 months he was walking with a cane. She is a single parent, trying to pay her bills, put her son though private college, and care for her chronically ill mother who lives with her. Thoughts of being unable to work are racing through her mind as she tries her best to focus on what the physician is saying. Areas of demyelination . . . Babinski's reflex . . . more tests like evoked potentials . . . sounds like he is speaking another language. She tries to look like she is following him, nodding as he continues but all she is thinking is that she wished she had thought to bring her sister with her. She didn't expect this at all.

The IOM (2004) stated that even "well-educated people with strong reading and writing skills may have trouble comprehending a medical form or doctor's instructions regarding a drug or procedure." In the above case scenario, the well-educated, highly experienced nurse is experiencing low health literacy. Health literacy is dependent upon the current context as well as previous knowledge base. Neurology is not her area of expertise and she was in a state of shock at the proposed working diagnosis. The physician thought he was individualizing the teaching to the experienced nurse but was unaware of her inability to understand the information he was explaining. She was too embarrassed to tell him she didn't understand and was overwhelmed. It can be easy to overestimate a patient's understanding of information or even not recognize a patient with low health literacy skills.

Theoretical/Conceptual Models

Although it is still challenging to define and measure health literacy, there has been a growing interest in related research. Health literacy has been the focus of the WHO, the Office of the U.S. Surgeon General, the IOM, the USDHHS,

The Joint Commission, the Agency for Healthcare Research and Quality, the AMA, the Centers for Medicare and Medicaid, and Healthy People 2010 and 2020. Despite being a national public health issue, there remains a lack of true theoretical frameworks that explain health literacy (Pleasant, McKinney, & Rickard, 2011). Without a common "gold standard" definition of health literacy and a foundational theory, it continues to be very difficult to research, measure, and progress the field of health literacy and ultimately enhance patient outcomes.

The Institute of Medicine (2004) provided two conceptual frameworks for health literacy. One placed literacy as the foundation of health literacy and health literacy as the central mediator between health contexts and individuals. In this framework health literacy served as the conduit between the individual's literacy skills and the health context (Figure 1.3). It also helps visualize the connection between health literacy and health outcomes.

The second framework illustrated by the IOM helps to visualize the interaction between and responsibility of three key sectors including cultural and societal factors, the education system, and the health care system (Figure 1.4).

This was not a causal representation, although the findings of limited health literacy and health outcomes do suggest a causal association. Conducting further research to demonstrate this association was suggested.

After review of the literature, the IOM committee concurred that the health system does not have sole responsibility for improvement in health literacy and that it is a shared responsibility among the three key sectors.

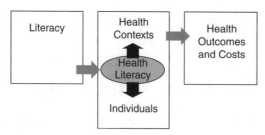

Figure 1.3 Health literacy framework.

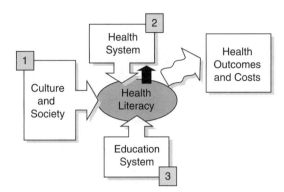

Figure 1.4 Potential points for intervention in the health literacy framework.

In addition, health literacy could be a determinant in explaining the established link between education and health.

One of the earlier concept analysis published in nursing by Speros (2005) reported an aim of assisting in defining the term health literacy as well as to clarify reference to it and also promote consistency in utilization of the concept in nursing and research. Defining attributes most often used in the literature were reading and numeracy skills, comprehension, using health information in decision making, and the ability to function in the role of a consumer of health care. Antecedents of health literacy were defined and included literacy as well as having a health-related experience. In addition, consequences of enhanced health were discussed and the role of nurses identifying consumers at high risk of low health literacy skills was emphasized.

Baker (2006) presented a conceptual model to define the domains of health literacy and the relationship of health literacy to health outcomes (Figure 1.5). It built upon the previous IOM report for a more specific discussion of the measures of health literacy.

The two major domains in Baker's models are individual capacity and health literacy. The individual capacity domain is further broken down into reading fluency, which is the ability to mentally process written information and gain new knowledge and prior knowledge, which includes vocabulary and a conceptual knowledge of health and health care (Baker, 2006). Baker further divided the health literacy domain into health-related oral literacy and health-related print literacy as was done in the IOM report. The measurement of new

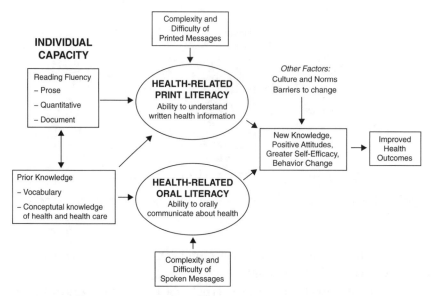

Figure 1.5 Conceptual model of the relationship between individual capacities, health-related print and oral literacy, and health outcomes.

knowledge, attitudes, and behaviors is represented in his model and is viewed as an outcome. Baker acknowledged that the majority of outcome measures were disease-specific knowledge and expressed the complexity of health literacy as a construct and the dependence upon a person's ability to communicate and the increasing demands of the health systems and society.

Paasche-Orlowe and Wolf (2007) emphasized a contextual appreciation of health literacy. Causal mechanisms of the health literacy–health outcomes relationship depend upon both the patient as well as the health care system. This conceptual model illustrates both individual and system factors that affect health care access, self-care, and the patient–provider encounter. Although this conceptual model illustrates a variety of interrelated critical occurrences such as social support, language, ethnicity, and age, Paasche-Orlow states the model has its limitations as it simplifies complex relationships.

In the concept analysis by Mancuso, the intricacies of health literacy are discussed. Mancuso refers to the "process of health literacy" (2008, p. 250) and that this process evolves over an individual's life span. As illustrated in Figure 1.6, the central attributes of health literacy are capacity, comprehension, and communication. The antecedents of health literacy encompass culture,

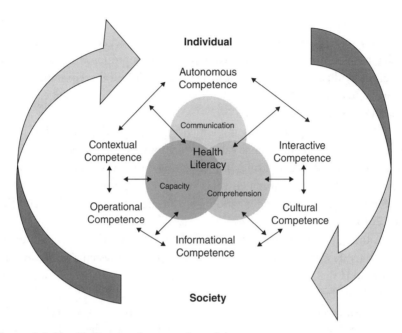

Figure 1.6 Health literacy: A concept model.

environment, language, learning together, sharing, and meaning of information. The skills of reading and understanding and language are inherent in the attributes of capacity and comprehension (Mancuso, 2008). Health literacy outcomes are dependent upon whether health literacy has been realized and also the potential to influence individuals and society.

Freedman describes limitations to the current definitions and conceptual models of health literacy as they "focus attention on and appear to limit the problem of health literacy to the capacity and competence of the individual" (Freedman et al., 2009, p. 446).

Health literacy is not an individual construct that starts and finishes with the patient. Another major limitation of several of the current conceptualizations is that the focus is on secondary and tertiary care rather than primary prevention of disease. In order to conduct health literacy research and change practice, Freedman states that social, political, environmental, and economic concerns must be included as they have an impact upon health. This change in focus would help in understanding and addressing societal level concerns that impact upon the public's health. A critical factor in transforming health care and the well-being of all individuals is the ability to truly engage patients in their care. Koh et al. (2013) propose a Health Literate Care Model that would ultimately weave health literacy strategies into all aspects of the Chronic Care Model, now known simply as the Care Model. This proposed model assumes that all individuals are at risk for low health literacy and therefore methods to confirm and ensure patient understanding would be incorporated at each point of care (Koh et al., 2013, p. 357).

Health care organizations implementing the model would align health literacy as a core organizational value throughout all components of strategic planning and the delivery of care. Implementing the Care Model with health literacy approaches could ultimately serve to reduce duplication and inefficiency while improving patient's understanding of and engagement in health care (Koh et al., 2013, p. 359).

Although further research is needed to demonstrate the impact of the Health Literate Care Model, it can represent a practical systems framework for organizations that aspire to adapt to the health literacy challenges of all individuals (Koh et al., 2013, p. 364).

Parnell describes the Health Literacy Tapestry (HLT) as a conceptual model (Figure 1.7) that emphasizes the fluidity of an individual's health literacy skills

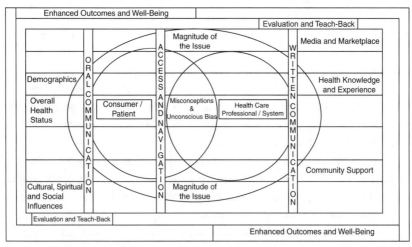

We should all know that diversity makes for a rich tapestry, and we must understand that all the threads of the tapestry are equal in value no matter what their color.

Maya Angelou

Figure 1.7 Health Literacy Tapestry.

dependent upon each specific health context. Tapestry is defined as "something felt to resemble a richly and complexly designed cloth" and is "used in reference to an intricate combination of things or sequence of events"(*American Heritage Dictionary*, 2012). This conceptual model uses a holistic nursing approach that is multidimensional, complex, nonstatic, with interwoven "threads" (antecedents) and "fibers" (domains) that impact upon both the individual and the system or provider factors. It represents the weaving of life experiences and behaviors with the health care system. The three basic "fibers" or domains include oral communication, written communication, and access and navigation. The skills associated with the stated "threads" may be cultivated, enhanced, or even diminish over time depending upon the life experience and specific context. The demographic thread includes race, ethnicity, age, and gender, while the thread representing health status incorporates vision, hearing, memory, and cognitive abilities. The remaining threads include previous health experience and knowledge, community support, cultural, spiritual, and social influences, and media and marketplace. This representation can be applied across the continuum of care, from acute to chronic care, with inpatient and ambulatory patients, through palliative and end-of-life care. Misconceptions and unconscious bias on both the part of the individual receiving care and the provider giving the care are central to the model. For example, limited English proficient patients have verbalized that they have refused interpreter services because they believed they had to pay for the service. We all have heard a professional express frustration about a patient not following a prescribed treatment plan and attribute it to their lack of caring or cooperation. Oftentimes, after further exploration it was disclosed that they could not afford the medication, didn't have transportation, or simply did not understand the treatment instructions provided. The HLT addresses the measurement of health literacy skills by the utilization of teach-back within each specific context. With the shift in health care to wellness and prevention, a health literacy conceptual model must be applicable to both wellness and illness. The HLT supports practices in health care, health promotion, and disease prevention. Therefore, the outcome measurement is prevention and enhanced well-being so that it can truly be applied across the life span and entire continuum of care. The tapestry is an accurate illustration of the need to develop true partnerships in the complex world of health literacy, health care, and individual health status. After all, enhancing health literacy is much more than understanding health information. It is also the complex task of empowering individuals to access, collaborate, navigate, and act upon the health information provided to enhance well-being.

The proposed HLT requires exploration and research to test the conceptual model. Perhaps initial research can apply the model to a specific disease state such as diabetes or hypertension. Research can also be done on a more global scale by applying the HLT to a wellness concept such as healthy behaviors or healthy lifestyles. There are a deficient number of nursing publications contributing to the research on nursing and health literacy. This conceptual model can serve as a catalyst to assist in the advancement of research and nursing theory that is applicable to the current demographic imperative and health care arena.

The nursing profession is ideally positioned to help consumers of health care cross the chasm between coverage and access as well as assist in the coordination of increasingly complex care. With more than 3 million members, the nursing profession represents the largest segment of the U.S. health care workforce (Census Bureau, 2009; Health Resources and Services Administration [HRSA], 2010) as cited in IOM (2011b, p. 23). Nursing practice covers the entire spectrum of health care, from health promotion, disease prevention, treatment of illness, coordination of care, to palliative and end-of-life care. Nurses play a crucial role throughout every aspect of this continuum, yet there is a lack of health literacy conceptual frameworks reported in the nursing literature. If nursing practice is based on nursing science we must continue to expand upon the development of conceptual frameworks for nursing research with the goal of enhancing nursing knowledge, guiding practice and ultimately enhancing patient outcomes.

Nursing Knowledge and Experience

Nurses are at the forefront of health care delivery and play a critical role in the promotion of health literacy thereby assisting in guiding our communities in reaching the overarching goal of The National Prevention Strategy to "increase the number of American's who are healthy at every stage of life" (National Prevention Council, 2011, p. 7). Teaching consumers of health care and health counseling are integral to nursing practice.

Nurses are employed across many areas of health care and public health, are true patient advocates, and are uniquely positioned to create a cultural change in health care that will shift the focus to optimizing health and wellness.

Richard Carmona, MD, MPH, FACS, the 17th Surgeon General of the United States, has often referred to "health literacy as the currency for success in everything we do in health, prevention and wellness." Yet, what is the health literacy knowledge and experience of our nursing colleagues? The majority of research on health literacy has historically focused on specific patient populations, acute versus chronic disease, and specific disease states, with less of a focus on the health literacy knowledge and experience of nurses.

The limited research results have unfortunately demonstrated that there are significant gaps among nurses regarding health literacy awareness, knowledge, skills, and practices that address low health literacy (Coleman, 2011; Cormier & Kotrlik, 2009). A study done by Mackert, Ball, and Lopez (2011) to improve information on the efficacy of a training program proposed to increase the health literacy knowledge of health professionals, demonstrated a marked improvement in the participants' perceived knowledge of health literacy. "A significant additional finding was the participants' overestimation of their own health literacy knowledge." Of note, the study did not measure the participants' behavior change as a result of the increased health literacy knowledge.

A Canadian pilot study of undergraduate nursing students integrating health literacy into the clinical setting (Zanchetta et al., 2012) reported several valuable results. The students valued their role as health educators and benefited both personally and professionally as their role expanded. One major theme that became apparent was their sensitivity to health literacy within a critical perspective. They demonstrated the ability to take a critical perspective and incorporate their clients' life contexts into the health teaching. Their clients were able to "harmonize the health information they gathered within their own cultural understanding of health and illness." The students' sensitivity to their clients' diversity enhanced the interconnectedness between health literacy and other social determinants of health. This training model is clearly representative of the positive outcomes that can occur when developing partnerships and providing patient-centered care.

Cormier and Kotrlik (2009) reported that knowledge gaps existed in the identification of older adults as a high-risk demographic for low health literacy. In addition, the senior baccalaureate nurses that participated in the research demonstrated a gap in the ability to screen for health literacy skills and assess guidelines for written patient education information.

Since continuing education activities require the identification of gaps in knowledge, health literacy should be incorporated as an integral component in all continuing nursing education activities. The provision of ongoing nursing education provides a wonderful opportunity and vehicle to address health literacy as well as the implications of low health literacy upon patient safety and patient outcomes.

Although it is encouraging to see that health literacy curricula for health care professionals are beginning to flourish, unfortunately there remains an absence of growth in these curricula reported in the nursing literature (Coleman, 2011). Nursing schools need to develop curricula and competencies to address this demonstrated gap in knowledge and skills. One of the goals of Healthy People 2020 is Health Communication and Health Information Technology with an objective to increase the health literacy skills of practitioners. Incorporating health literacy throughout the curricula will help ensure that our future nurses are adequately prepared to provide patient-centered care, improve health care outcomes, and eliminate disparities in care.

Health Literacy Resources for Nurses

Books

Bastable, S. B. (2006). *Essentials of patient education.* Sudbury, MA: Jones & Bartlett.

Doak, C. C., Doak, L. G., & Root, J. H. (1996). *Teaching patients with low literacy skills* (2nd ed.). Philadelphia, PA: J.B. Lippincott.

Jeffreys, M. R. (2010). *Teaching cultural competence in nursing and health care.* New York, NY: Springer Publishing Company.

Marks, R. (2012). *Health literacy and school-based health education.* Bingley, West Yorkshire, UK: Emerald Group Publishing Limited.

Nielsen-Bohlman, L., Panzer, A., Hamlin, B., & Kindig, D. A. (Eds.). (2004). *Health literacy: A prescription to end confusion.* Washington, DC: The National Academies Press.

Osborne, H. (2004). *Health literacy from A to Z: Practical ways to communicate your health.* Sudbury, MA: Jones & Bartlett.

Schwartzberg, J. G., et al. (2005). *Understanding health literacy: Implications for medicine and public health.* Chicago, IL: American Medical Association.

Schwartzberg, J. G. (2003). *Health literacy: Help your patients understand.* Chicago, IL: American Medical Association.

Reports

The National Assessment of Adult Literacy (NAAL). *America's health literacy: Why we need accessible health information.* Retrieved from http://health .gov/communication/literacy/issuebrief

Health literacy: A prescription to end confusion. Institute of Medicine, Washington, DC: The National Academies Press. Retrieved from http://www.iom .edu/Reports/2004/Health-Literacy-A-Prescription-to-End-Confusion.aspx

IOM Roundtable on Health Literacy: The mission of the Roundtable is to advance the field of health literacy by translating research findings into practical strategies that can be implemented. To achieve this mission, the Roundtable discusses challenges facing health literacy practice and research, and identifies approaches to promote health literacy in the public and private sectors. *Visit this site to access the many IOM reports on health literacy.* Retrieved from http://www.iom.edu/Activities/PublicHealth/HealthLiteracy.aspx

Office of the U.S. Surgeon General 2006. *Proceedings of the Surgeon General's Workshop on Improving Health Literacy, National Center for Biotechnology Information, U.S. National Library of Medicine.* This report summarizes presentations on the state of health literacy from a variety of perspectives, including those of health care organizations and providers, the research community, and educators. Retrieved from http://www.ncbi.nlm.nih.gov/books/NBK44257

Websites

The Agency for Healthcare Research and Quality (AHRQ)—www.ahrq.gov/qual/literacy

American Academy of Ambulatory Nurses (AAACN)—www.aaacn.org

American Medical Association Foundation—Health Literacy Kit—www.ama-asn.org

Centers for Disease Control and Prevention (CDC)—www.cdc.gov/healthliteracy

Centers for Disease Control and Prevention (CDC) Plain Language Thesaurus—www.plainlnaguage.gov/populartopics/health_literacy/index.cfm

Harvard School of Public Health—www.hsph.harvard.edu/healthliteracy/resources

Health Resources and Services Administration (HRSA)—www.hrsa.gov

National Action Plan to Improve Health Literacy—www.healthgov/communication/hlactionplan

The Joint Commission—www.jointcommission.org

- 2007—Hospitals, Language and Culture—A Snapshot of the Nation
- 2007—What Did the Doctor Say?: Improving Health Literacy to Protect Patient Safety
- 2008—One Size Does Not Fit All: Meeting the Health Care Needs of Diverse Populations
- 2010—Advancing Effective Communication, Cultural Competence, and Patient and Family Centered Care . . . A Roadmap for Hospitals

The Joint Commission—Speak Up to Prevent Errors in Your Care
—www.jointcommission.org/speakup.aspx

National Network of Libraries of Medicine (NNLM)—www.nnlm.gov

The Plain Language Action and Information Network (PLAIN)
—www.plainlanguage.gov

References

Ad Hoc Committee on Health Literacy. (1999). Health literacy: Report of the Council on Scientific Affairs. *JAMA, 281*, 552–557.

American heritage dictionary of the English language, fourth edition. (2012). Retrieved from http://www.wordnik.com/words/tapestry

American Medical Association. (2005). *Understanding health literacy: Implications for medicine and public health.* Chicago, IL: AMA Press.

Baker, D. W. (2006). The meaning and measure of health literacy. *Journal of General Internal Medicine, 21*, 878–883.

Berkman, N. D., Davis, T. C., & McCormack, L. (2010). Health literacy: What is it? *Journal of Health Communication, 15*, 9–19.

Castro, C. M., Wilson, C., Wang, F., & Schillinger, D. (2007). Babel babble: Physicians' use of unclarified medical jargon with patients. *American Journal of Health Behavior, 31*(Suppl. 1), S85–S95.

Centers for Disease Control and Prevention. (2010). Retrieved from http://www.cdc.gov/healthliteracy/Learn

Coleman, C. (2011). Teaching health care professionals about health literacy: A review of the literature. *Nursing Outlook, 59*, 70–78.

Cormier, C. M., & Kotrlik, J. W. (2009). Health literacy knowledge and experiences of senior baccalaureate nursing students. *Journal of Nursing Education, 48*(5), 237–248.

Cutilli, C. C., & Bennett, I. M. (2009). Understanding the health literacy of America. Results of the National Assessment of Adult Literacy. *Orthopaedic Nursing, 28*, 27–32.

Doak, C. C., Doak, L. G., & Root, J. H. (1996). *Teaching patients with low literacy skills* (2nd ed.). Philadelphia, PA: JB Lippincott Company.

Freedman, D. A., Bess, K. D., Tucker, H. A., Boyd, D. L., Tuckman, A. M., & Wallston, K. A. (2009). Public health literacy defined. *American Journal of Preventive Medicine, 336*, 446–451.

Goodman, M., Finnegan, R., Mohadjer, L., Krenzke, T., & Hogan, J. (2013). *Literacy, numeracy, and problem solving in technology-rich environments among U.S. adults: Results from the Program for the International Assessment of Adult Competencies 2012: First look (NCES 2014-008).* U.S. Department of Education. Washington, DC: National Center for Education Statistics. Retrieved from http://nces.ed.gov/pubsearch

Institute of Medicine. (2011a). *Promoting health literacy to encourage prevention and wellness: A workshop summary.* Washington, DC: The National Academies Press.

Institute of Medicine. (2011b). *The future of nursing: Leading change, advancing health,* Washington, DC: The National Academies Press.

Koh, H., Brach, C., Harris, L. M., & Parchman, M. L. (2013). A proposed 'Health Literate Care Model' would constitute a systems approach to improving patients' engagement in care. *Health Affairs,* No. 2, 357–367.

Kutner, M., Greenberg, E., Jin, Y., & Paulson, C. (2006). *The health literacy of America's adults: Results from the 2003 National Assessment of Adult Literacy (NCES 2006-483).* U.S. Department of Education. Washington, DC: National Center for Education Statistics.

Mackert, M., Ball, J., & Lopez, N. (2011). Health literacy awareness training for healthcare workers: Improving knowledge and intentions to use clear communication techniques. *Patient Education and Counseling, 85,* e225–e228.

Mancuso, J. M. (2008). Health literacy: A concept/dimensional analysis. *Nursing Health Sciences, 10,* 248–255.

McCabe, J. A. (2006). An assignment for building an awareness of the intersection of health literacy and cultural competence skills. *Journal of the Medical Library Association, 94,* 458–461.

Murphy-Knoll, L. (2007). Low health literacy puts patients at risk. The Joint Commission update. *Journal of Nursing Care Quality, 22,* 205–209.

National Prevention Council. (2011). *National prevention strategy,* Washington, DC: U.S. Department of Health and Human Services, Office of the Surgeon General.

Nielsen-Bohlman, L., Panzer, A., Hamlin, B., & Kindig, D. A. (Eds.). (2004). *Health literacy: A prescription to end confusion.* Washington, DC: The National Academies Press.

Nutbeam, D. (2000). Health literacy as a public goal: A challenge for contemporary health education and communication strategies into the 21st century. *Health Promotion International, 15,* 259–267.

Organisation for Economic Co-operation and Development. (2012). *Literacy, numeracy, and problem solving in technology-rich environments: Framework for the OECD survey of adult skills, OECD Publishing.* Retrieved from http//www.oecd-ilibrary.org/education/literacy-numeracy-and-problem-solving-in-technology-rich-environments_9789264128859.en

Paasche-Orlow, M. K., & Wolf, M. S. (2007). The causal pathways linking health literacy to health outcomes. *American Journal of Health Behavior, 31* (Suppl. 1), S19–S26.

Parikh, N. S., Parker, R. M., Nurss, J. R., Baker, D. W., & Williams, M. V. (1996). Shame and health literacy: The unspoken connection. *Patient Education and Counseling, 27,* 33–39.

Pleasant, A., McKinney, J., & Rickard, R. (2011). Health literacy measurement: A proposed research agenda. *Journal of Health Communication, 16* (Suppl. 3), 11–21.

Ratzan, S. C. (2001). Health literacy: Communication for the public good. *Health Promotion International, 16,* 207–214.

Ratzan, S. C., & Parker, R. M. (2000). Introduction. In C. R. Selden, M. Zorn, S. C. Ratzan, & R. M. Parker (Eds.), *National Library of Medicine current bibliographies in medicine: Health literacy.* Bethesda, MD: National Institutes of Health, U.S. Department of Health and Human Services.

Sorensen, K., Broucke, S. V., Fullam, J., Doyle, G., Pelikan, J., Slonska, A., & Brand, H.; HLS-EU Consortium Health Literacy Project European. (2012). Health literacy and public health: A systematic review and integration of definitions and models. *BMC Public Health, 12,* 80. doi:10:1186/1471-2458-12-80

Speros, C. (2005). Health literacy: Concept analysis. *Journal of Advanced Nursing, 50,* 633–640.

U. S. Department of Education. (2003). National Center for Education Statistics. *The health literacy of America's adults: Results from the 2003 National Assessment of Adult Literacy.* Retrieved from http://nces.ed.gov/pubsearch/pubsinfo.asp?pubid=2006483

U.S. Department of Education. (2012). National Center for Education Statistics, Organisation for Economic Co-operation and Development (OECD). Program for the International Assessment of Adult Competencies (PIAAC).

U.S. Department of Health and Human Services, O.D.P.H.P. (2000). Health communication objective. *Healthy People, 1*(11), 11.1–11.27.

U.S. Department of Health and Human Services. (2010). Retrieved from www .healthypeople.gov

Weiss, B. D. (2007). *Health literacy and patient safety: Help patients understand.* Chicago, IL: American Medical Association.

White, S. (2008). *Assessing the nation's health literacy: Key concepts and findings of the National Assessment of Adult Literacy (NAAL).* Chicago, IL: American Medical Association Foundation.

White, S., & McCloskey, M. (forthcoming). *Framework for the 2003 National Assessment of Adult Literacy (NCES 2005-531).* U.S. Department of Education. Washington, DC: National Center for Education Statistics.

World Health Organization. (1998). *Division of Health Promotion, Education and Communications Health Education and Health Promotion Unit. Health promotion glossary.* Geneva, Switzerland: Author.

Zanchetta, M., Taher, Y., Fredericks, S., Waddell, J., Fine, C., & Sales, R. (2012). Undergraduate nursing students integrating health literacy in clinical settings. *Nurse Education Today, 33*(9), 1026–1033.

Zarcadoolas, C., Pleasant, A., & Greer, D. (2005). Understanding health literacy: An expanded model. *Health Promotion International, 20,* 195–203.

Low Health Literacy and Implications

Terri Ann Parnell

M r. George is a 51-year-old Caucasian male that many describe as a high-powered businessman. He owns his own commercial real estate business and is always working. Even on his days "off" he is always "on." As he says, "It's my business, I have to be accessible. If not it could mean losing a huge deal!" Over the past few weeks, he has been feeling more fatigued, and has had a few episodes of "achiness" down his left arm. He has attributed it to beginning to exercise again and his strenuous workout at the gym and the corporate tennis match he just participated in. After 2 solid weeks of "just not feeling himself" he decided to go to his primary care physician. He was also tired of hearing his wife insist that he "should go to the doctor to get checked out" on a daily basis.

After a physical exam, blood work, and a stress test, his physician wanted him to have an elective cardiac catheterization. The procedure seemed to go well. After his recovery period, his doctor came to his room and told him that to his surprise his "catheterization results were positive for blockages and that he will need a few more tests before he sees him in his office to discuss his treatment plan."

Low health literacy remains a crosscutting priority in health care that places many individuals at risk who cannot understand and act upon the information needed to receive quality health care. As illustrated in the National Assessment of Adult Literacy (NAAL) Report (see Chapter 1, Figure 1.2), 36%

or over 75 million adults had basic or below basic health literacy. If these data applied to a communicable disease, a solution would be integrated across the entire continuum of care for all individuals entering the health care system. Unfortunately, we still have many opportunities to enhance strategies for health literacy improvement.

Additional research suggests that low health literacy skills can be applicable to persons of all literacy levels. Why do we as health care professionals assume everyone can understand the language we speak? At first glance, most would agree that a college-educated businessman who owns his own commercial real estate company is an "educated consumer" of health care. However, when his physician enters his room to tell him that his "test results are positive and that he will need a few more tests" before he sees him in the office, the businessman immediately calls his wife to say, "Honey, I have good news. Dr. Smith said my test results were positive and I just need some more tests before I go back to his office." In this situation positive really meant that the results were not favorable. Yet, why do we assume that consumers of health care will know when positive is reflective of a good result or a bad result.

Low health literacy will affect most adults at some point throughout their lifetime. Therefore it is key for all health care providers to keep health literacy as a vital component when caring for patients of any age, culture, education, or socioeconomic status (Berkman et al., 2004). In fact, health literacy has been referred to as the "currency" for improving the quality of U.S. health, health care, and health outcomes (Paasche-Orlow, Parker, Gazmararian, Nielsen-Bohlman, & Rudd, 2005). As Dr. Richard Carmona MD, MPH, FACS, and 17th Surgeon General of the United States has said, "Health literacy is the currency for success in everything we do. In search of the holy grail for health care, we can no longer afford to keep health literacy on the sidelines."

Low Health Literacy Implications: Consumers of Health Care

Health consumers face growing health literacy challenges as they attempt to access, navigate, and understand the increasingly complex health care system. In addition, there is the increasing burden of chronic disease management, the need to engage as 50-50 partners in their care, and the abundance of health information available from numerous and often conflicting sources. Individuals are now asked to assume expanded roles in seeking information, advocating for their rights and privacy, understanding responsibilities, measuring and monitoring their own health and that of their community, and making decisions about insurance and care options (Institute of Medicine [IOM], 2004).

The health consumers that will be most affected by low health literacy are those with less education, low socioeconomic status, the elderly, and those that experience cultural and linguistic barriers. However, even those with advanced education and financial means are struggling to keep up with the new roles and responsibilities expected of them as they attempt to engage in this new health care arena. The growing complexity of health care and the focus on consumer-driven health plans, medical and flexible accounts, complex prescription plans, self-disease management, and shared decision making are burdens to many. In fact, many consumers of health care feel intimidated and overwhelmed by the complexity of the system and do not want to participate in shared decision making. The most capable and caring nurse cannot encourage a healthy lifestyle or enhance a patient's health outcome alone. Patients must be partners in their care and their health literacy skills, and the degree of patient engagement can have an impact upon their health outcomes.

Obtaining Health Information

Health literacy skills and health information needs can vary greatly from one consumer to another as well as for the same consumer depending upon the current context. Health information can be communicated in many ways. One method is through written materials such as brochures, fact sheets, posters, prescription labels, and consent forms. Many consumers prefer to seek out health information electronically, whether from a DVD or CD, on a website, or via email, tweets, and interactive blogs. There is also interpersonal communication, the "old standby" that some consumers still feel most comfortable with. They prefer speaking with their health care providers and the office staff to assist with access, navigation, and obtaining health information. In addition, consumers also obtain health information from television, books, magazines, newspapers, and the Internet.

Changes in technology and more immediate expectations of many consumers have led to an increase in use of technical resources for health information. In a recent survey by PricewaterhouseCoopers, 54% of consumers used online tools and resources second to consulting with a physician (75%) when gathering information on treatments and conditions. In addition, individuals seek health care information from third-party media and information service companies three and a half times more than any other online health information source (PricewaterhouseCoopers, 2010, p. 18). Another survey reported that about 93 million Americans have searched for at least one of 16 major health topics online (Fox & Fallows, 2003). These findings show an increase in the number of individuals who are considered "health seekers." Online health seekers are primarily women and they tend to search for information on a specific diagnosis, prescription, preparing for and recovering from surgery, and caregiver tips. However, there are often gaps in and misunderstanding of the health information available to consumers. Much of the health information accessed can be written in a very complex way at a reading level that often exceeds the individual's reading ability (Rudd, Moeykens, & Colton, 2000). For individuals with low health literacy, the challenge of obtaining, understanding, and applying the information to change behavior or make informed decisions can be quite challenging.

Health consumers with limited literacy, cognitive, and language skills may find websites an even greater challenge to navigate. Most importantly, many consumers searching the Internet are unaware of how to determine if the information being provided is quality, evidence-based health information. One initiative to help improve the quality and the ability for consumers to understand health information is the Plain Writing Act of 2010 (see Chapter 5, The Tipping Point). This act required federal agencies to use plain language in government communication including health information (The Plain Language Writing Act, 2010).

Most people at some point in their life will be responsible for caring for an aging parent or relative. Our population is aging and in the year 2000, people ages 65 and older represented 12.4% of the U.S. population but by 2030 are now expected to represent 19% of the population (Administration on Aging, 2013). In addition, many adults are living with chronic illness and this trend will be compounded as the adult population continues to age. The National Academy for an Aging Society estimates that $73 billion in unnecessary health care costs can be attributed to inadequate health literacy due to misunderstood information and subsequent patient noncompliance (Center for Health Care Strategies, 2000).

Numerous studies have shown that the management of these complex chronic illnesses often falls upon family members or friends as caregivers (Reinhard, Levine, & Samis, 2012). Being a caregiver is independently associated with health-related activities and the health literacy skills of the caregiver. It has been reported that 39% of U.S. adults provide care for a loved one, up from 30% in 2010, and many navigate health care with the help of technology (Fox, Duggan, & Purcell, 2013). Caregivers often look for resources to assist them with their ability to cope with the stress associated with caregiving. Caregivers have a tremendous responsibility and often try to quickly gather complex health information and make decisions regarding care. An aging population and more adults living with chronic illnesses will translate into an increase in family caregivers' accessing, deciphering, and making decisions based upon online health information.

It is becoming increasingly common to ask patients to schedule appointments, refill prescriptions, and even ask questions they may have for their health care provider through online technology. Universal health information technology is also a central focus of health care reform. In a study to assess the use of an industry-leading patient portal, clear racial, ethnic disparities in patient portal use were demonstrated as well as differences in educational attainment. Much lower rates of patient portal use were reported among those with limited health literacy as compared to those with adequate health literacy (Sarkar et al., 2010). As health care reform continues to focus on health information technology, health literacy, education, and racial disparities will exist in the use of patient portals.

Informed Consent

Although informed consent in the patient care setting is not just about the content that is actually written on the consent form and having the patient sign it, having this informed discussion and formal signature establishes a difference between informed consent and patient education (Fleisher, n.d., para. 2). Informed consent in the patient care setting occurs when the health care professional informs the patient of risks, benefits, and alternatives to the procedure or treatment so that the patient can make an informed, knowledgeable decision about care. The consequences of not fully understanding the informed consent process can be devastating.

Health literacy plays a vital role in the informed consent process, in regard to both the written document and the verbal conversation. Most consent forms are very long and complex, incorporating unexplained medical terminology, or are text dense, poorly formatted with small font size, and have very high reading levels. In a U.S. medical school survey, grade level readability for informed consent documents were between a 5th-grade to 10th-grade readability level (Paasche-Orlow, Taylor, & Brancati, 2003). According to the IOM, "the readability levels of informed consent documents (for research and clinical practice) exceed the documented average reading levels of the majority of adults in the United States" (IOM, 2004, p. 191). The implications of this have not been fully researched, yet most would agree that they are far reaching.

In addition to the written document for review and signature, a discussion must occur between the health care professional and patient to share information regarding the risks, benefits, and alternatives to the procedure or treatment. The information should be provided in a way the patient can understand to be certain that the patient can effectively make an informed decision. The Joint Commission and the Centers for Medicare and Medicaid (CMS) emphasize education and training specific to the patient's abilities and patient involvement when obtaining an informed consent. The informed consent conversation should ideally be a collaborative decision-making discussion that incorporates the patient's beliefs, culture, religion, language, and education level, and should not be only about obtaining a signature on a form. Those in the health literacy field are very well aware of the often-told story shared by a woman who was a poor reader, when she went to the gynecologist office for a problem and unknowingly signed the surgical consent for a hysterectomy. The physician referred to her surgery as "an easy repair," she asked no questions, and scheduled the surgical date. She did not realize it until she came back for her post surgical checkup and the nurse asked her "How are you feeling after your hysterectomy?" (Cordell, 2007).

Health care professionals have a responsibility to enhance the informed consent process. Several methods can be incorporated such as writing consent forms at a lower reading level by incorporating plain language, providing health literate patient education materials, incorporating the use of visual aids, and, if possible, allowing for time between the informed consent discussion and the procedure or surgery. The National Quality Forum identifies teach-back when obtaining informed consent as a top safety practice (National Quality Forum, 2010). Incorporating teach-back after the discussion to ensure that patients are able to repeat back in their own words what was explained would be very beneficial.

Medication Management

When a patient goes to the clinic, emergency department, hospital, or doctor's office, it is common to leave with either a prescription for medication or instructions for obtaining over-the-counter medication. Communication about medications, especially medications with the potential of serious consequences if taken incorrectly, are considered high-risk situations.

The implications between low health literacy and medication management has been well documented. Research studies have shown a link between low health literacy and misunderstanding of prescription medication instructions leading to medication errors. In fact, adults with low health literacy experience more serious medication errors compared to persons with adequate health literacy (Schillinger et al., 2005) and limited health literacy was deemed a barrier to patients' taking hypertension medication (Persell, Osborn, Richard, Skripkauskas, & Wolf, 2007).

At first glance, prescription labels may appear to list quite simple instructions, yet they are often unclear and very confusing to consumers. The prescription often incorporates a variety of written and pictorial information about the drug label and drug warnings. To further complicate proper administration, if there is a medication device (cup, dosing spoon, or dropper) included for dosing, it is often very difficult to read and is sometimes not compatible with the dosage instructions. Yin et al. (2010) reported that dosing errors by parents were highly prevalent with cups as compared to droppers, spoons, or syringes and suggested that strategies to reduce errors should address both the use of the dosing device and health literacy.

Over the past 10 years, Americans who took at least one prescription drug in the past month increased from 44% to 48%. The use of two or more drugs increased from 25% to 31% and the use of five or more drugs increased from 6% to 11% (Gu, Dillon & Burt, 2010). Among older Americans aged 60 and over, more than 76% used two or more prescription drugs and 37% used five or more (Figure 2.1).

Polypharmacy, or the use of multiple medications in Americans aged 60 and over, is increasingly becoming a serious issue for both consumers and

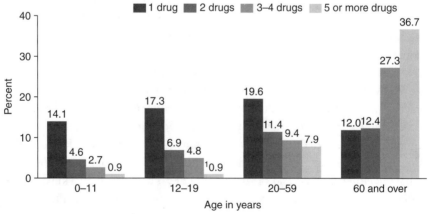

¹Estimate is unstable; the relative standard error is greater than 30%.
Source: CDC/NCHS, National Health and Nutrition Examination Survey.

Figure 2.1 Percentage of prescription drugs used in the last month, by age: United States, 2007–2008.

providers in the health care system. It has been reported that patients 65 years old and older are the largest consumers of both prescription and over-the-counter medications in the United States and significant morbidity and mortality are associated with inappropriate polypharmacy (Bushardt, Massey, Simpson, Ariail, & Simpson, 2008).

Effective communication about medications and prescription use is a key aspect of following prescribed therapies. In addition, there are many other skills needed when deconstructing the activity of taking a prescribed medication. As noted by researcher Dr. Rima Rudd from the Harvard School of Public Health, deconstructing the health activity includes the delineation of all associated tasks, identifying the literacy skills needed for each individual task, and identifying the tools and then the skills needed for each tool. Deconstructing the health activity will assist in determining the overall literacy demand (Harvard School of Public Health, 2013).

For example, when deconstructing the activity of properly taking medication there are many tasks. These may include taking the prescription to the pharmacy, picking up the medication, checking if the prescription is correct, reading the label, comprehending the information, speaking with the pharmacist if necessary, and signing to accept or decline information from the pharmacist. For each of these tasks, there are associated tools and skills a person needs to use, many focused on reading, comprehension, and numeracy. When taking the single task of reading the prescription label, the skills that are needed can include comprehending the name of the medication, understanding the dosage or strength, the number of times each day to take, when to take the medication, how many pills to take, number of refills, and understanding any specially colored warning labels and instructions. The skills necessary become even more complex as more and more medications are added, each containing different instructions.

The goal of a recent study by Wolf et al. (2011) of 464 adults (average age 63.3 years) who were receiving care either at an academic general medicine practice or at one of three federally qualified health centers was to evaluate the accuracy and variability in the way patients would schedule a typical seven-drug regimen. They reported that most participants (71.1%) were female and highly educated (61.4% were college graduates); however, nearly half were identified as having either low (20.7%) or marginal (22.8%) health literacy skills. It concluded that many patients do not consolidate prescriptions in an efficient way, which can affect safe adherence.

As patients with low health literacy are at greater risk of incorrectly taking their medications, the authors propose a universal medication schedule of morning, noon, evening, and bedtime to assist in standardizing the prescribing

practices of practitioners. Additional research needs to be conducted to establish the evidence needed to support this suggestion. Other areas of concern
requiring additional research related to polypharmacy, health literacy, and the
hospitalized patient are the use of the electronic medication order entry and
medication reconciliation.

Implementation of the Affordable Care Act and Health Insurance Exchanges

In 2014, millions of people are expected to have access to health insurance coverage. The Patient Protection and Affordable Care Act (ACA) aims to decrease
the number of uninsured Americans and improve the quality of care provided
while containing health care costs. There is tremendous uncertainty during
this unfamiliar and very critical time in health care in the United States. The
ACA will expand access to it for many people who may be obtaining it for the
very first time. There will be state and federal health insurance exchanges and
expanded Medicaid subsidies to choose from. This comes with a tremendous
burden for many new consumers of health care. Consumers will need adequate
health literacy skills to interpret and understand the new changes, their options,
and the cost of the choices they select. However, since low health literacy tends
to be more prevalent in persons with low socioeconomic status, low educational status, and minority groups, most of the newly eligible persons will also
most likely have low health literacy skills (Rudd, Anderson, Oppenheimer, &
Nath, 2007). In addition, with the implementation of the ACA, more limited
English proficient persons (LEP) will have access to health insurance and health
care services.

The cognitive burden upon the newly insured will be quite high. Enrollment
choices in a health insurance plan are considered a complex task (Dorn, 2011).
What actually is health insurance, who is the subscriber and provider, what is a
dependent or beneficiary, how to decide who is in network or out-of-network
is just the beginning of a new language that will need extensive explanation.
When explaining this new concept of health insurance, and all of the components within it, one must be certain that the consumer is able to teach-back the
meaning and concepts in his or her own words. When explaining health insurance it can be helpful to use analogies and individualize the explanation to the
consumer. For example, a comparison between health insurance and car insurance can be quite helpful. Car insurance protects against unanticipated financial
loss such as an accident but does not pay for routine care and expenses such as

an oil change. Health insurance helps pay for the routine care and "check-ups" such as screenings and also helps pay for high cost expenses (Patel et al., 2013).

Consumers will also be faced with understanding how to enroll and once covered, how to use health insurance. Interpreting what services are and are not covered, the previsit paperwork, and what documents are necessary to bring to each health care encounter are essential for access and navigation. Cost is also a vital consideration when purchasing health insurance. Consumer cost sharing, premiums, deductibles, and co-payments are terms and concepts that are complicated to understand. Four questions (Patel et al., 2013) that can assist consumers when enrolling in a new health insurance plan are:

1. What are my choices for health insurance?

2. How do I get it?

3. How do I use it?

4. How much will it cost me?

While the ACA does not focus specifically on health literacy, successful implementation will be affected by efforts focused on enhancing strategies to ensure that consumers understand, know how to access and use the insurance, and are fully aware of the financial costs of participation.

Chronic Disease Management

The epidemic of chronic illness, which represents 75% of the $2 trillion in annual U.S. health care spending, is steadily moving toward crisis proportions (IOM, 2012). Chronic diseases such as heart disease, stroke, cancer, diabetes, and arthritis are among the most common, costly, and preventable diseases in the United States. Seven out of 10 American deaths each year are from chronic diseases with heart disease, cancer, and stroke accounting for more than 50% of all deaths each year (Kung, Hoyert, Xu, & Murphy, 2008). As a nation, 75% of our health care dollars goes to treatment of chronic diseases (Centers for Disease Control and Prevention [CDC], 2013).

Patients with low health literacy and chronic illness have extremely complex management needs. When patients cannot understand their instructions or cannot remember directions provided, management of their chronic disease is more difficult for both the patient and health care professional. There is increased responsibility now being placed upon the patient for self-monitoring of signs and symptoms and overall condition. They must know when to adjust their treatment, know when to call and who to call to report more serious information to their health care professional. These are highly skilled tasks requiring a proficient level of health literacy and often the tasks that are most overwhelming to patients when managing their chronic illnesses.

The heightened collaboration that is necessary among the patient, health care professional, health care system, and community to enhance patient outcomes adds an extra dimension of complexity to the care provided to persons with chronic disease. Chronic disease exemplifies the interaction of health literacy and health, as patient health outcomes are often dependent upon the patient's ability and willingness to follow a set of health activities essential to the management and treatment of chronic disease (IOM, 2004, p. 171). Enhancing collaborative efforts among health care systems, public health, and the community can assist in enhancing prevention and treatment outcomes for persons living with and managing chronic disease.

Low Health Literacy Implications: Providers of Health Care and Health Care Systems

Low health literacy also places health care providers and the health care system at risk. Narrowing the gap that exists between the health literacy skills of persons receiving care and the professionals or systems providing the care would help enhance patient outcomes and overall patient safety. Research has demonstrated that clinicians have a tendency to underestimate the information needs of their patients (Cegala, 1997) and in the clinical setting tend to overestimate the health literacy of their patients (Ryan et al., 2008). It is imperative that nurses and health care professionals take an active role in closing the gap that exists between the providers and receivers of health information.

Unconscious Bias

Nurses can enhance an individual's health literacy skills by taking a moment to pause and reflect upon their own unconscious biases and the impact this can have upon effective communication, patient-centered care, patient safety, and patient outcomes. You may be surprised at this statement and actually be thinking, "That's not true. I don't have any biases and I take good care of all my patients regardless of who they are." However, unconscious bias among all health care professionals can contribute to health disparities. In the IOM report, *Unequal Treatment* (Smedley, Stith, & Nelson, 2003), it was reported that unrecognized bias against certain racial or ethnic minorities may actually affect communication or the care that is offered to these persons.

In *Seeing Patients: Unconscious Bias in Health Care*, White (2011) suggests that there is subconscious disparity being practiced by physicians. He identified 13 groups of patients that experience health care discrimination or disparities and many of these identified groups are also similar to the individuals that also experience low health literacy. They are not only the racial, ethnic, or religious groups that one typically thinks of when discussing disparities in health care, but also include women, the obese, the elderly, the disabled, and prisoners. The professionals with unconscious bias are not malicious or bad practitioners, but rather, are most often well-meaning. They just do not have any idea about how their subconscious thoughts can have such an impact upon communication, diagnosis, and treatment options.

Unconscious bias can occur without a person's intent or even realizing it is occurring and, therefore, controlling it can be a difficult matter. Since we all have some bias of one kind or another, beginning with self-awareness is one way all health care professionals can begin to lessen their bias. This is especially true of nurses who are their patients' gatekeepers and advocates. Nurses make decisions every day that can have an impact upon patient safety and outcomes, and unconscious bias influences each of these patient provider interactions.

Patients and caregivers should also be aware that unconscious bias exists. White (2011) advised patients to increase their health literacy and knowledge of their illness and condition and to be polite but forthright with their health care provider about bias if they feel they are experiencing it.

Financial Implications

Health literacy should always be the foundation for all that we plan and do in health care now as well as with the implementation of health care reform. Low health literacy impacts a person's health and it also has tremendous financial impact on the individual, the health care system, and the public. There are many factors that contribute to the increased cost of health care for providers and the health care system. Studies have reported that there is a correlation between individuals with low health literacy and poor health outcomes (Berkman et al., 2004). Hospital admissions, physician visits, medication management, home health care, and nursing home services, along with the rising increase in chronic disease, all contribute to this increased cost of care. In a study of primary care patients who were asked about their understanding of medications, treatment options, cause of their diagnosis, and their confidence managing their health condition, results indicated that patients who are more confident in their ability to manage their care and who understand their treatment choices cost approximately 8% less to treat than those with less knowledge about their health (Hibbard, Greene, & Overton, 2013).

Persons with low health literacy incur increased medical costs to the health care system. In fact, research has shown that inpatient spending for a patient with inadequate health literacy was $993 higher than that of a patient with adequate reading skills (Baker et al., 2002). In addition, persons with low health literacy are more likely to make medication errors, have more difficulty navigating the health care system, are less likely to follow medical treatments, and more likely to be hospitalized (IOM, 2004).

There are nearly $90 million adults in the United States with low health literacy. Although low health literacy is a crosscutting priority for adults of all ages, races, ethnicities, education levels, and linguistic abilities, low health literacy is disproportionately higher among those of less socioeconomic status, less education, or those with limited English proficiency. This is also true of older adults and those with physical and mental disabilities (IOM, 2011a). With the launch of the ACA in 2014, millions of Americans are expected to be covered by health insurance, many for the very first time. Many of the individuals obtaining health insurance for the first time will be the least prepared to realize the benefits due to low health literacy (IOM, 2011a). Under the ACA, more persons who are limited English proficient (LEP) will have health insurance and need to obtain services in their preferred language. LEP patients have increased rate of readmission, longer lengths of stay, and are at a higher risk of poorer health outcomes. The financial impact for caring for LEP patients is higher due to the potential complications that can arise from language barriers, as well as the inefficient use of health care services. Developing a language and communication access plan with policies and procedures, properly training all staff, and implementing a comprehensive language interpretation service are necessary to achieve quality care for LEP patients.

In addition, as reimbursement shifts from a fee-for-service delivery system toward an outcomes-based system, providers and hospitals are looking for new ways to transform the delivery of health care. Many hospitals and health care systems are forming partnerships with physician groups, urgent-care centers, and ambulatory clinics in an effort to offer less expensive, more convenient quality health care.

It is difficult for health care providers and health care systems to predict who will participate in the ACA, what their needs will be, and what resources will be necessary to manage their medical needs. The goals of the implementation of the ACA will not be reached unless the health literacy skills of both individuals and the health care system are addressed (IOM, 2011a). The combination of low health literacy, an aging patient population, self-management of chronic disease, and the increased difficulty accessing and navigating a very complicated system places additional financial burden on the United States health care system.

Low Health Literacy Implications: Beyond the Health Care System

Educational System

There are many opportunities to introduce health literacy throughout the United States educational system. Incorporating consistent and coordinated health literacy education and activities early in childhood will help prepare children to reduce risky health-related behaviors and live a healthy lifestyle. The U.S. educational system offers a primary point of intervention to improve the quality of both literacy and health literacy. In its report on health literacy, the IOM found that "achieving health literacy in students is hindered by a lack of continuity in health education programs across the many age groups" (IOM, 2004, p. 143).

In a study by the CDC, it was reported that most elementary, middle, and high schools require health education classes as part of the curriculum (Kann, Brenner, & Allensworth, 2001). The majority of the states use the National Health Education Standards (NHES), which describe the knowledge and skills needed for health literacy and health education by the end of grades 2, 5, 8, and 12 (CDC, 2007). They were initially published in 1995, revised in February 2007, and continue to be the accepted roadmap for health education in school systems (Table 2.1).

The standards have a focus on personal health and wellness and emphasize the integration of social and behavioral sciences. Each of the eight standards

Table 2.1 National Health Education Standards

Standard 1	Students will comprehend concepts related to health promotion and disease prevention to enhance health.
Standard 2	Students will analyze the influence of family, peers, culture, media, technology, and other factors on health behaviors.
Standard 3	Students will demonstrate the ability to access valid information and products and services to enhance health.
Standard 4	Students will demonstrate the ability to use interpersonal communication skills to enhance health and avoid or reduce health risks.
Standard 5	Students will demonstrate the ability to use decision-making skills to enhance health.
Standard 6	Students will demonstrate the ability to use goal-setting skills to enhance health.
Standard 7	Students will demonstrate the ability to practice health-enhancing behaviors and avoid or reduce health risks.
Standard 8	Students will demonstrate the ability to advocate for personal, family, and community health.

touches on the development of health literacy skills. They incorporate accessing health information and care, prevention and management of illness, goal setting and advocacy. The implementation of health education and the National Health Education Standards in the schools can be enhanced when they become integrated as part of the overall school health program and can be reinforced by other projects, initiatives, and components.

Although most schools require this education, inconsistency and a lack of coordinated effort exist when building upon the foundational knowledge learned in the prior years. Kann et al. (2001) also reported that the percentage of schools requiring students to take health education decreased as the grade level advanced, from 27% in grade 6, 20% in grade 8, 10% in grade 9, and 2% in grade 11. This lack of a coordinated approach hinders achieving health literate students and ultimately health literate adults.

The Education for Health Framework builds upon health literacy, undergraduate public health and evidence-based practice, which are areas that have recently been developed or have experienced significant growth (Riegelman, 2010). It builds upon these nationally acknowledged movements in an effort to create a cogent education strategy that can build upon the foundation

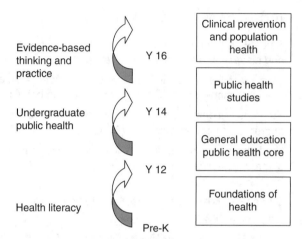

Figure 2.2 Education for Health Framework designed to connect the educational phases to achieve Healthy People 2020 objectives.

that has been laid and ensure measureable outcomes. The Education for Health Framework (Figure 2.2) aims for a vertical approach across age groups as well as horizontal integration among educators, clinicians, and public health practitioners and was designed as educational roadmap for Healthy People 2020 (Riegelman & Garr, 2011).

Population health, wellness, and prevention are crucial areas to encourage collaboration across professions. Although the health literacy effort began to assist consumers in a health care environment, it has increasingly become part of personal health and wellness activities aligning with the educational system.

Adult Literacy

The field of adult education, inclusive of general education development (GED), adult basic education (ABE), and English for speakers of other languages (ESOL), provides a wonderful opportunity for aligning common synergies and enhancing the health literacy of adult learners. Enhancing partnerships between adult educators and health care professionals can help students apply the basic skills learned to a health context and enhance their ability to become healthy citizens. This collaboration is often overlooked as adult educators are not experts in the field of medicine and health care professionals are not experts in developing curricula and applying learning principles. However, the adult educators do not need to be experts in health if they shift their focus to teaching the adult learners the skills that are necessary to apply to health care situations. By using this skills-based approach, it has teachers identify the common connections between the skills, the students are already learning with what they will need to do for their health (Soricine, Rudd, Santos, & Capistrant, 2007). Many common health-related tasks such as filling out demographic intake forms, wayfinding in a health care building, selecting what foods are appropriate for a specific prescribed diet, or recalling and reporting personal past medical history can be difficult for all. However for adults that are learning English or obtaining their GED, it can be even more daunting and overwhelming.

According to Soricine et al. (2007), the skills-based approach has similar goals but different roles in health literacy. For example, the health care professional might teach a patient how to use an asthma inhaler and the adult educator may teach the student to ask questions about tests, procedures, and devices. Another example of shared goals but different roles cited by Soricine is the health care professional prescribing medication and explaining the reason for taking it and its potential side effects, and the adult educator teaching the student how to read the medication label, schedule the proper timing of the prescribed regimen, and calculate the proper dosage.

There are many areas that can be linked when integrating health literacy skills in adult education. When teaching basic reading, writing, math, and communication skills, linkages can be made to enhance health literacy skills related to these areas. For example, when the adult educator is teaching about disease prevention, one area of focus may be that adults are expected to be able to determine risk and engage in preventive screenings. Skill-based tasks to assist with this lesson plan can be incorporated into reading articles in newspapers, numeracy skills when looking at and interpreting charts and graphs, and communication skills when discussing follow-up care after a screening.

Adult educators are valuable resources that can enhance health literacy skills of adult learners. They are already teaching the everyday skills needed to function in society, and can incorporate the same skills into the health-related items such as prevention, wellness, and disease management. Using a skills-based approach to integrate health literacy into adult education will create a learning environment that allows the students to take what was learned and transfer those basic skills into all that they experience in society and ultimately become a health literate consumer of health care.

Culture, Language, and Community Partnerships

Integrating health literacy into community partnerships is crucial given the changing ethnic, religious, and linguistic demographics of the United States. For these increasingly diverse communities, culture and language determine the lens through which individuals apply health literacy skills. Culture defines how one feels about health and illness and also how, when, and from whom a person seeks out health care. It can also impact how individuals follow a pre-scribed treatment plan and how they respond and adapt to behavior and life-style changes. Culture provides the context and meaning that is gained from information, as well as the purpose by which people come to understand their health status, diagnosis, and treatment plan (IOM, 2004).

Different cultures also have varying ways of communicating, including words, body language and gestures, and what is appropriate to be discussed and with whom. It is not uncommon for words or the meaning of the words to vary from culture to culture. The promotion of health literacy in different cultures and communities necessitates the provision of providing patient- and family-centered care with an awareness of the potential differences in meaning. Culture is not static but rather a fluid process for individuals and communities. It is imperative to understand that even communities with similar cultures consist of people and families with multiple beliefs and backgrounds and they should not be placed into a stereotypical box by using ethnic and linguistic labels that can have a negative impact upon patient safety and outcomes. Nurses need the agility to seamlessly move from the familiarity of their own cultural beliefs and values to the culture of their patient. Health literacy skills are intertwined within the cultural and linguistic skills of each patient.

Speaking and listening are examples of health literacy skills that are influenced by both culture and language. Limited English proficiency is a definite barrier to a patient's ability to effectively listen and speak. Even with the provision of a qualified medical interpreter to assist in effective communication, there can still be cultural issues that may interfere with the effectiveness of communication between the patient and health care professional (Singleton & Krause, 2009).

Numeracy skills are very important when selecting health insurance, discussing treatment options, making health care decisions, managing medication regimens, and interpreting lab and test results. Imagine the story of a mother from a culture that does not use spoons, who reads a medication label that states to give her child one teaspoon of medicine. She uses a large soup spoonful of the medicine rather than a teaspoon because it was their custom to use chopsticks and soup spoons for meals (Andrulis & Brach, 2007). The mother was not familiar with the many sizes of spoons available and therefore gave her child too much medicine.

Decision making is another health literacy skill that is influenced by culture and language. Nurses may assume that a patient is responsible for making his or her health decisions, however, in certain cultures it may be the most senior male family member who makes the decisions for all in the family. This may be viewed as inappropriate or incorrect to the American nurse caring for the patient. Patients must make decisions that are congruent with their cultural beliefs and traditions. Therefore it is important that nurses consider the patient's cultural and religious beliefs when discussing treatment or discharge instructions to avoid conflict and noncompliance with the prescribed regimen.

Partnering with our communities is crucial to enhance mutual understanding of each other's cultures and beliefs. Community members and health care professionals need to collaborate to learn from each other, enhance effective communication, and foster a relationship of dignity and respect. This partnership will ultimately enhance the provision of patient-centered care, enhance patient safety, and improve overall health care outcomes.

Low Health Literacy Implications: A Public Health Issue

Traditionally, the focus of public health has been on the social and environmental determinants of health. More recently, there has been a shift on this focus to include the modification of individual risk behaviors toward prevention and wellness. As the focus of providing health care is shifting to include a prevention and wellness model, health literacy must evolve to also be integrated into activities outside of the health care system. The IOM (1988) has defined public health as "fulfilling society's interest in assuring conditions in which people can be healthy." Health literacy remains a crosscutting priority that impacts upon all health care efforts across the entire spectrum from prevention to illness and from birth through each stage of life. In 2011, The ACA called for the development of the National Prevention Strategy to achieve the benefits of prevention for all Americans' health. The overarching goal of the National Prevention Strategy is to increase the number of Americans who are healthy at every stage of life (National Prevention Council, 2011, p. 7). Preventing disease and injuries is key to the improvement of Americans' health and many of the strongest predictors of health and wellness fall outside of the health care setting (National Prevention Council, 2011, p. 6). Public health is not only defined by health care but also by what people do each day outside the system (IOM, 2011b).

The incorporation of many diverse partners is necessary to achieve such an ambitious goal. Examples of such partners may include businesses and employers, faith-based organizations, educational facilities such as early learning centers, schools, technical programs, and colleges, as well as community organizations.

A person with adequate health literacy is able to take full responsibility for his or her own health, the health of the family, and the community (McQueen, Potvin, Pelikan, Balbo, & Abel, 2007). The IOM report (2004) states that health literacy is a shared function of social and individual factors, which emerges from the interaction of the skills of individuals and the demands of social systems. The medical perspective on factors influencing people's health should be shifted toward a societal level. Public health literacy can be found when the conceptual foundations of health literacy are placed in a group or community (Freedman et al., 2009). Health literacy has a direct impact upon health behavior and therefore impacts upon health outcomes and on health care costs in society. From a public health lens, a health literate person is able to fully participate in his or her health care. The benefits of health literacy have a tremendous impact on all activities of daily living including activities at home, the workplace, and in society. Advancing health literacy will empower individuals, bring us to more equity, and help to sustain changes in the public health arena.

Health literacy remains a crosscutting priority that impacts all health care efforts across the entire spectrum from prevention to wellness and illness. With the changing demographics and changing ways of delivering health care, health literacy continues to be a critical issue that requires integration into all prevention, wellness, and illness models. As nursing professionals, we have a tremendous responsibility to provide health information in an understandable, action-oriented way that will facilitate the empowerment of individuals to improve their health as well as the health of their communities and society at large.

References

Administration on Aging. (2013). *Aging statistics*. Department of Health and Human Services. Retrieved June 25, 2013, from http://www.aoa.gov/Aging_Statistics

Andrulis, B., & Brach, C. (2007). Integrating literacy, culture, and language to improve health care quality for diverse population. *American Journal of Health Behavior, 31*, S122–S133.

Baker, D. W., Gazmararian, J. A., Williams, M. V., Scott, T., Parker, R., Green, D., . . . Peel, J. (2002). Functional health literacy and the risk of hospital admission among Medicare managed care enrollees. *American Journal of Public Health, 92*(8), 1278–1283.

Berkman, N. D., DeWalt, D. A., Pignone, M. P., Sheridan, S. L., Lohr, K. N., Lux, L., . . . Bonito, A. J. (2004). *Literacy and health outcomes. Evidence Report/Technology Assessment No. 87* (prepared by RTI International–University of North Carolina Evidence-based Practice Center under Contract No. 290-02-0016). AHRQ Publication No. 04-E007-2. Rockville, MD: Agency for Healthcare Research and Quality.

Bushardt, R. L., Massey, E. B., Simpson, T. W., Ariail, J. C., & Simpson, K. N. (2008). Polypharmacy: Misleading but manageable. *Clinical Interventions in Aging, 3*(2), 383–389.

Cegala, D. J. (1997). A study of doctors' and patients' communication during a primary care consultation: Implications for communication training. *Journal of Health Communication, 2*(3), 169–194.

Center for Health Care Strategies. (2000). *CHCS fact sheets. Facts about health literacy: Low health literacy skills increase annual health care expenditures by $73 billion.* Princeton, NJ: Center for Health Care Strategies.

Centers for Disease Control and Prevention. (2007). *National Health Education Standards—Achieving excellence.* Retrieved June 25, 2013, from http://www .cdc.gov/healthyyouth/sher/standards/index.htm

Centers for Disease Control and Prevention. (2013). *Chronic disease prevention and health promotion.* Retrieved August 26, 2013, from http://www.cdc .gov/chronicdisease/index.htm

Cordell, T. (2007). Chasing the monster. *North Carolina Medical Journal, 68*(5), 331–332.

Dorn, S. (2011). *Implementing national health reform: A 5-part strategy for reaching the eligible uninsured.* Washington, DC: Urban Institute.

Fleisher, L., et al. (n.d.). *A practical guide to informed consent.* Retrieved from http://www.templehealth.org/ICTOOLKIT/html/ictoolkitpage27.html

Fox, S., Duggan, M., & Purcell, K. (2013). Internet Health Resources, Pew Internet & American Life. *Family caregivers are wired for health.* Retrieved June 25, 2013, from http://pewinternet.org/Reports/2013/Family-Caregivers.aspx

Fox, S., & Fallows, D. (2003). Internet Health Resources, Pew Internet & American Life Project. Retrieved June 25, 2013, from http://www.pewinternet.org

Freedman, D. A., Bess, K. D., Tucker, H. A., Boyd, D. L., Tuchman, A. M., & Wallston, K.A. (2009). Public health literacy defined. *American Journal of Preventative Medicine, 36*(5), 446–451.

Gu, Q., Dillon, C. F., & Burt, V. L. (2010). *Prescription drug use continues to increase: U.S. prescription drug data for 2007–2008.* NCHS data brief, no 42. Hyattsville, MD: National Center for Health Statistics.

The Harvard School of Public Health: Health Literacy Studies Website. Retrieved July 31, 2013, from http:www.hsph.harvard.edu/healthliteracy

Hibbard, J. H., Greene, J., & Overton, V. (2013). Patients with lower activation associated with higher costs; delivery systems should know their patients' scores. *Health Affairs, 32,* 2216–2222.

Institute of Medicine. (1988). *The future of public health.* Washington, DC: The National Academies Press.

Institute of Medicine. (2004). *Health literacy: A prescription to end confusion.* Washington, DC: The National Academies Press.

Institute of Medicine. (2011a). *Health literacy implications for health care reform: A workshop summary.* Washington, DC: The National Academies Press.

Institute of Medicine. (2011b). *Promoting health literacy to encourage prevention and wellness: Workshop summary.* Washington, DC: The National Academies Press.

Institute of Medicine. (2012). *Living well with chronic illness: A call for public health action.* Washington, DC: The National Academies Press.

Kann, L., Brener, N. D., & Allensworth, D. D. (2001). Health education: Results from the School Health Policies and Programs Study 2000. *Journal of School Health, 71*(7), 266–278.

Kung, H. C., Hoyert, D. L., Xu, J. Q., & Murphy, S. L. (2008). Deaths: Final data for 2005. *National Vital Statistics Reports, 56*(10), 1–120.

McQueen, D., Potvin, L., Pelikan, J. M., Balbo, L., & Abel, Th. (Eds.). (2007). *Health and modernity: The role of theory in health promotion.* New York, NY: Springer.

National Prevention Council. (2011). *National prevention strategy.* Washington, DC: U.S. Department of Health and Human Services, Office of the Surgeon General.

National Quality Forum. (2010). *Safe practices for better health care—2010 update.* Washington, DC: National Quality Forum.

Paasche-Orlow, M. K., Parker, R. M., Gazmararian, J. A., Nielsen-Bohlman, L. T., & Rudd, R. R. (2005). The prevalence of low health literacy. *Journal of General Internal Medicine, 20*(2), 175–194.

Paasche-Orlow, M. K., Taylor, H. A., & Brancati, F. L. (2003). Readability standards for informed consent forms as compared with actual readability. *New England Journal of Medicine, 348,* 721–726.

Patel, K. K., West, M. L., Hernandez, L. M., Wu, V. Y., Wong, W. F., & Parker, R. M. (2013). *Helping consumers understand and use health insurance in 2014.* Discussion Paper. Washington, DC: Institute of Medicine. Retrieved from http://iom.edu/Global/Perspectives/2013/HelpingConsumersUnderstandUse HealthInsurance.aspx

Persell, S. D., Osborn, C. Y., Richard, R., Skripkauskas, S., & Wolf, M. S. (2007). Limited health literacy is a barrier to medication reconciliation in ambulatory care. *Journal of General Internal Medicine, 22,* 1523–1526.

PricewaterhouseCoopers. (2010). *Top health industry issues of 2011.* New York, NY: Author.

Reinhard, C., Levine, C., & Samis, S. (2012). *Alone: Family caregivers providing complex chronic care.* AARP Public Public Policy Institute and the United Hospital Fund. Retrieved June 25, 2013, from http://www.aarp.org/ home-family/caregiving/info-10-2012/home-alone-family-caregivers-providing-complex-chronic-care.html

Riegelman, R. (2010). Education for health: An educational underpinning for Healthy People 2020. *Public Health Reports, 125,* 148–152.

Riegelman, R. K., & Garr, D. R. (2011). Healthy People 2020 and education for health. What are the objectives? *American Journal of Preventive Medicine, 40*(2), 203–206.

Rudd, R., Anderson, J., Oppenheimer, S., & Nath, C. (2007). Health literacy: An update of public health and medical literature. In J. Comings, B. Garner, & C. Smith (Eds.), *Review of adult learning and literacy* (Vol. 7, pp. 174–204). Mahwah, NJ: Lawrence Erlbaum Associates.

Rudd, R. E., Moeykens, B. A., & Colton, T. C. (2000). Health and literacy: A review of medical and public health literature. In J. P. Comings, B. Garner, & C. Smith (Eds.), *The annual review of adult literacy and learning.* Mahwah, NJ: Lawrence Erlbaum Associates.

Ryan, J. G., Leguen, F., Weiss, B. D., Albury, S., Jennings, T., Velez, F., & Salibi, N. (2008). Will patients agree to have their literacy skills assessed in clinical practice? *Health Education Research, 23*(4), 603–611.

Sarkar, U., Karter, A. J., Liu, J. Y., Adler, N. E., Nguyen, R., Lopez, A., & Schillinger, D. (2010). The literacy divide: Health literacy and the use of an internet-based patient portal in an integrated health system—Results from the Diabetes Study of Northern California

(DISTANCE). *Journal of Health Communication; International Perspectives, 15*(Suppl. 2), 183–196.

Schillinger, D. E., Machtinger, L., Wang, F., Chen, L. L., Win, K., Palacios, J., . . . Bindman, A. (2005). *Language, literacy, and communication regarding medication in an anticoagulation clinic: Are pictures better than words? Advances in patient safety: From research to implementation.* Rockville, MD: Agency for Healthcare Research and Quality.

Singleton, K., & Krause, E., (2009). Understanding cultural and linguistic barriers to health literacy. *OJIN: The Online Journal of Issues in Nursing, 14*(3), Manuscript 4.

Smedley, B. D., Stith, A. Y., & Nelson, A. R., (Eds). (2003). *Unequal treatment: Confronting racial and ethnic disparities in health care.* Washington, DC: The National Academies Press.

Soricine, L., Rudd, R., Santos, M., & Capistrant, B. (2007). *Health literacy in adult basic education. Designing lessons, units, and evaluation plans for an integrated curriculum.* Boston, MA: National Center for the Study of Adult Learning and Literacy; Health and Adult Literacy and Learning Initiative. Harvard School of Public Health.

The Plain Language Writing Act. (2010). *Improving communication from the federal government to the public.* Public law 111–274, 11th Congress. Retrieved June 25, 2013, from http://www.plainlanguage.gov/plLaw

White, A. (2011). *Seeing patients: Unconscious bias in health care.* Cambridge, MA: Harvard University Press.

Wolf, M. S., Curtis, L. M., Waite, K., Bailey, S. C., Hedlund, L. A., Davis, T. C., . . . Wood, A. L. (2011). Helping patients simplify and safely use complex prescription regimens. *Archives of Internal Medicine, 171*(4), 300–305.

Yin, H. S., Mendelsohn, A. L., Wolf, M. S., Parker, R. M., Fierman, A., van Schaick, L., . . . Dreyer, B. P. (2010). Parents' medication administration errors: Role of dosing instruments and heath literacy. *Archives of Pediatrics & Adolescent Medicine, 164*(2), 181–186. doi:10.1001/archpediatrics.2009.269

3

Delivering Patient-Centered Care in a Diverse Environment

Jennifer H. Mieres

A patient is an individual to be cared for, not a medical condition to be treated. Our patients are our partners and have knowledge that is essential to their care. Patient-Family Centered Care is the core of a high-quality healthcare system and a necessary foundation for safe, effective, timely and equitable care. (Cooper University Health Care, 2013)

As the diversity of the United States continues to grow, the health care community will increasingly encounter patients with innumerable languages and cultures. Recent evidence demonstrates a strong link between a person's culture and the perception of health problems, the meaning and understanding of health problems, the communication of health problems, and ultimately health outcomes. Therefore, for the delivery of safe and quality health care, health care systems must customize health care delivery methods to incorporate cultural health care beliefs so as to meet the growing needs of increasingly diverse and multicultural populations. This chapter focuses on the importance of and the incorporation of health literacy as a component in cultural and linguistic proficiency in the delivery of quality patient-centered care to diverse populations. A clinical case is presented to facilitate a discussion of the components of patient-centered care. An expanded approach to the delivery of health care to include health care team education and curriculum expansion for health care professionals is presented. The importance of the Patient Protection and Affordable Care Act (ACA) in the elimination of health care disparities, the link with the delivery of safe quality patient care to culturally customized care, and the integration of effective communication with a focus on health literacy are discussed.

Importance of Linking the Delivery of Safe, Quality Patient Care to Culturally Customized Patient-Centered Care

In 2001, the Institute of Medicine (IOM) published the groundbreaking report *Crossing the Quality of Chasm*, which identified patient-centeredness as an essential foundation for quality and patient safety. This landmark publication issued a call to action for a reorientation of the health care delivery system to a holistic approach, whereby the delivery of health care centered on the needs of the patient is considered equally as important as the care itself. This patient-centered care approach does not replace exceptional medicine; it both complements clinical excellence and contributes to it through effective partnerships and communication (IOM, 2001).

In the broadest terms, patient-centered care is care that is structured around the patient. It is a model in which the health care team partners with patients and families to identify and satisfy the full range of patient needs and preferences.

Several years ago, the Picker Institute published eight principles of patient centered care, which embody Picker's conviction that all patients deserve high-quality health care and that patients' views and experiences are integral to achieving excellent health outcomes. The principles of patient-centered care are: (1) respect for patients' values, preferences, and expressed needs; (2) coordination and integration of care; (3) information, communication, and education; (4) physical comfort; (5) emotional support and alleviation of fear and anxiety; (6) involvement of family and friends; (7) transition and continuity; and (8) access to care (Frampton et al., 2008).

For the effective delivery of safe, quality, and excellent patient-centered care, health care professionals, health care teams, and health care systems must adopt and integrate into clinical practice an expanded cross-cultural approach to culturally competent clinical practice. This approach must focus on awareness of crosscutting cultural and social issues, health beliefs that are present in all cultures, and communication skills (Saha, Beach, & Cooper, 2008, p. 1277).

Effective communication is a critical component of the delivery of safe quality patient-centered care and, as such, health literacy is critical to the improvement of health and wellness (Benjamin, 2010). As per the recent U.S. Department of Health and Human Services (USDHSS) report, the cultural and linguistic differences among patients directly impact their health literacy levels, which, in turn, is a contributing factor to an increased prevalence of health disparities among racial and ethnic minorities, immigrants, low-income individuals, and nonnative speakers of English and elderly adults (Hasnain-Wynia & Wolf, 2010, p. 897; U.S. Surgeon General and USDHHS, 2007).

Clinical Case Scenario

MJ, a 72-year-old Haitian woman, arrived by emergency medical service to the emergency department (ED) of her local hospital with complaints of 4 days of abdominal pain and sudden syncope. She was accompanied by her 45-year-old daughter. Upon arrival to the hospital, she was awake and alert, appeared agitated, speaking in French and Creole. The triage nurse quickly began to get a history and soon discovered that MJ did not understand what was happening and that getting a history would be challenging, as MJ did not speak English as she alternated between speaking French and Creole. MJ was quickly placed in a room and the nurse quickly took vital signs and continued to try to get a history as MJ's daughter who spoke French, Creole, and broken English served as the translator. The ED physician was quickly called to the room, as MJ's began writhing in pain and had evidence of gastrointestinal bleeding. As it became evident that MJ may need to have emergency abdominal surgery, her daughter panicked, with MJ becoming agitated and very upset as her daughter explained to her in Creole that surgery may be needed. The surgical team had arrived and without realizing that MJ did not speak English as a first language, began telling her about the surgical procedure needed for her diverticulitis and requested her consent for the procedure. MJ became more agitated and her daughter had to interrupt the surgeon to let him know that MJ did not understand as English was not her primary language.

Over the next 6 hours, there was a delay in diagnosis and treatment of MJ as she and her daughter refused surgery and refused the required imaging studies due to lack of communication and MJ's fears of abdominal surgery. Later that night at the change of staff shift, a Haitian nurse was assigned to MJ and was able to speak to MJ and her daughter in Creole and alleviated MJ's cultural fears about abdominal surgery, explained these fears to the surgical team, and gained the trust of MJ and her daughter. MJ had successful surgery for diverticulitis the next day and was discharged 10 days later.

Applications of Patient-Centered Principles to the Case Scenario

The health care team's only focus in dealing with MJ centered around making a diagnosis and establishing a treatment strategy. There was an underrecognition of the fact that effective health communication is as important to health care as the clinical skill of establishing a diagnosis and treatment strategy. Two of the Picker principles of patient-centered care are applicable in dealing with MJ and her daughter: (1) respect for patients' values, preferences, and expressed needs, and (2) integration of information, communication, and education. There was a complete lack of recognition for the importance of health literacy and failure to request an interpreter who would have taken the burden of interpretation from MJ's daughter. An interpreter would have been able to communicate MJ's cultural fears of abdominal surgery as well as her personal fears of abdominal surgery as she had lost two family members during abdominal surgery in Haiti. In addition, an appreciation and understanding of the Haitian cultural beliefs about illness (i.e., Haitians have a fatalistic view of illness, reflected in the expression, "God is good," and great fear of abdominal surgery) would have helped the surgical team in gaining the trust of MJ and her family (Colin & Paperwall, 2003, p. 535).

MJ's case underscores the importance of the critical factors in the delivery of safe, quality, patient-centered care, the incorporation of beliefs, values, traditions, and practices of a culture, and culturally based belief systems of the etiology of illness and disease and those related to health and healing.

Culture and the Link to Health Care

The delivery of high-quality health care that is accessible, effective, and safe requires all health care practitioners and the entire health care team to have a deeper understanding of the sociocultural background of patients, their families, and the environments in which they live. There is a need of education and a comprehensive understanding of the word "culture." An understanding that culture comprises a myriad of variables, affecting all aspects of experience, is essential. Recognition that cultural practices frequently differ within the same ethnic or social group because of differences in age among generations, gender, religion, political association, class, ethnicity, and even personality is important in patient-centered care. The health care team needs to acknowledge that a multicultural approach to cultural competence can result in stereotypical thinking rather than clinical competence (Saha, Beach, & Cooper, 2008, p. 1279). The expanded cross-cultural approach to culturally competent clinical practice, which focuses on foundational communication skills, awareness of crosscutting cultural and social issues, and health beliefs that are present in all cultures, must be adopted and integrated into all aspects of health care delivery. We can think of these as universal human beliefs, needs, and traits (National Center for Cultural Competence, 2010). This patient-centered approach relies on identifying and negotiating different styles of communication, decision-making preferences, roles of family, sexual and gender issues, and issues of mistrust, prejudice, and racism, among other factors. The evidence supports the fact that culturally competent health care services facilitate clinical encounters with more favorable outcomes, enhance the potential for a more rewarding interpersonal experience and increase the satisfaction of the individual receiving health care services (Goode, Dunne, & Bronheim, 2006).

Critical factors in the provision of culturally competent health care services include understanding of the beliefs, values, traditions, and practices of a culture; culturally defined health-related needs of individuals, families, and communities; culturally based belief systems of the etiology of illness and disease and those related to health and healing; and attitudes toward seeking help from health care professionals (National Center for Cultural Competence, 2010).

Therefore, in any clinical encounter and for the accurate diagnosis and the establishment of a treatment plan, the health care team must understand the beliefs that shape a person's approach to health and illness. Knowledge of customs and healing traditions are indispensable to the design of treatment and interventions for diverse populations (Goode, Dunne, & Bronheim, 2006).

There is a compelling need for all health care systems, hospitals, and members of the medical team to become culturally competent whereby competence means having the capacity to function effectively as individuals and an organization within the context of cultural beliefs, behaviors, and needs presented by the members and their communities.

The integration of the tenets of cultural competency defined as the "ability of systems to provide care to patients with diverse values, beliefs and behaviors, including tailoring delivery to meet patients' social, cultural and linguistic needs" into health care systems and into the clinical encounter is essential for the delivery of health care to diverse populations (Health Research & Educational Trust, July 2011). As per the National Center for Cultural Competence (2010), culturally competent health care systems acknowledge and incorporate into the daily fabric all aspects of quality of care metrics: (1) importance of culture; (2) assessment of cross-cultural relations; (3) recognition of potential impact of cultural differences; (4) expansions of cultural knowledge; (5) adaption of services to meet culturally unique needs; (6) increased diversity of workforce and leadership; (7) strategies to promote diversity in all hiring and recruitment; and (8) assessment of bias, stereotypes, and prejudice in organizational and leaders' behaviors (Health Research & Educational Trust, July 2011).

Cultural and Linguistic Competence in the Delivery of Patient-Centered Care

As immigration to the United States continuously expands our nation's demographic composition, and the make up of the American population has expanded to include racially, ethnically, culturally, and linguistically diverse populations, there is a need for the health care community to meet the health needs of a diverse population (Shrestha & Heisler, 2011, p. 28). Minority groups are the fastest growing demographic, currently accounting for one third of the U.S. population (Betancourt et al., 2012).

Immigration has had a significant influence on the size and age structure of the U.S. population. By 2043, racial and ethnic minorities are projected to account for a majority of the U.S. population (Health Research & Educational Trust, 2013). According to the U.S. Census 2000 Supplementary Survey of U.S. households, the number of Americans who do not speak English has soared over the past decade (Pandya, Batalova, & McHugh, 2011). Approximately 25 million people in the United States (8.6%) are defined as limited English proficient (LEP) and are therefore at risk for adverse events because of language and cultural barriers. LEP individuals tend to have higher rates of hospital readmission, longer lengths of stay, and greater medical complications (Betancourt et al., 2012).

Recognition of the fundamental differences among people from various nationalities, ethnicities, and cultures, and the affect on health beliefs is important for members of the health care community (National Center for Cultural Competence, 2010). Applying the Picker Institute's eight principles of patient-centered care for a diverse population requires the inclusion of cultural competence to ensure care is individualized and equitable and there is a focus on the development of multidisciplinary programs to improve the patient-centeredness and cultural competence of health professionals (Frampton et al., 2008)

In making a diagnosis, the health care team must understand the beliefs that shape a person's approach to health and illness. Knowledge of customs and healing traditions are indispensable to the design of treatment and interventions (National Center for Cultural Competence, 2010). Effective health communication is as important to health care as clinical skill. To improve individual health and build healthy communities, health care providers need to recognize and address the unique culture, language, and health literacy of diverse communities (National Center for Cultural Competence, 2010). Critical factors in the provision of culturally competent health care services include understanding of the (1) beliefs, values, traditions and practices of a culture; (2) culturally defined, health-related needs of individuals, families, and communities; (3) culturally based belief systems of the etiology of illness and disease and those related to health and healing; and (4) attitudes toward self. Therefore, there is a compelling need for all health care systems, hospitals, and members of the medical team to become culturally competent whereby competence means having the capacity to function effectively as individuals and an organization within the context of cultural beliefs, behaviors, and needs presented by the members and their communities (Betancourt, Green, & Carrillo, 2002).

Given the fact that in the United States greater than 55 million people speak a language other than English and that culture and language influence the health, healing, and wellness belief systems, as well as how illness, disease, and their causes are perceived, there is a critical need for the integration of cultural and linguistic competence in all aspects of health care delivery. Cultural beliefs also affect the behaviors of patients who are seeking health care and their attitudes toward health care providers and the health care team. Ultimately, the delivery of services by a health care team who are not culturally sensitive and who are incapable of effective communication can compromise access for patients from other cultures (National Center for Cultural Competence, 2010).

Figure 3.1 illustrates the necessary components for organizational achievement of cultural and linguistic competence. The four components, (1) Community Data Collection, (2) Humanism, (3) Communication and Language Access Services, and (d) Health Literacy, are all integral to the achievement of cultural and linguistic competence (Cross et al., 1989).

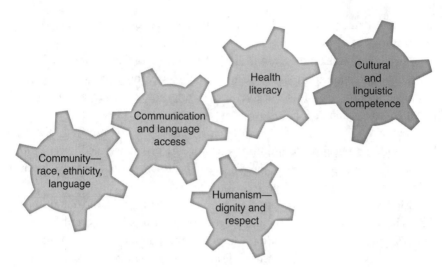

Figure 3.1 Components for cultural and linguistic competence.

Adapted from Cross et al. (1989).

Community Data: Importance of Collection of Race, Ethnicity, and Language

Before a health care organization becomes culturally competent, leaders must understand the local community and the role the organization plays within the community. A partnership with the community in the journey for community health and wellness must be established (Figure 3.1). Therefore, health care systems must build a community coalition and collect and analyze data to understand the health care needs including language and other needs so as to improve health care delivery services for the local community. A focused approach on educating the health care team and alignment of programming and resources to meet community health needs is essential for the delivery of safe, quality care. The collection of race, ethnicity, and language (REAL) data is a necessary first step to understanding the health care needs of the populations served. Obtaining feedback on performance on quality measures across patient population and developing appropriate quality improvement interventions with data standardization are of critical importance for ensuring the delivery of culturally and linguistically appropriate care. The ability to identify disparities and monitor efforts to reduce them has been limited due to a lack of specificity, uniformity, and quality in data collection and reporting procedures (Smedley, Stith, & Nelson, 2009). As stated by the IOM, consistent methods for collecting and reporting health data by race, ethnicity, and language are essential to informing evidence-based disparity-reduction initiatives, such as those that address variations in quality of care or facilitate the provision of culturally and linguistically appropriate services (Ulmer, McFadden, & Nerenz, 2009).

Improvements in data collection and reporting by race, ethnicity, and language have the potential to enhance the evidence-base for new health care improvement strategies for diverse communities, and, additionally, to raise awareness about the persistence of health disparities (Betancourt et al., 2012).

Humanism

Incorporating tenets of humanism whereby everyone is treated with dignity and respect will foster an inclusive health care culture leading to better relationships with patients and communities. This approach ultimately can result in the provision of care that is compassionate and high quality, incorporating diverse values, beliefs, and behaviors and ensuring that the delivery of care meets the patient's social, cultural, and linguistic needs (Frampton et al., 2008).

Communication and Language Services

The integration of communication, language, and interpreter services is essential to the delivery of care that is culturally and linguistically appropriate as health care is significantly compromised if we cannot communicate with diverse communities in which English is a second language and with the hearing or visually impaired. Lack of effective communication with patients and their families will impair the ability to collect information to establish diagnostic and treatment strategies, obtain informed consent for required treatment and procedures, develop relationships and trust, discuss treatment options, and provide necessary health care education. Lack of effective communication, secondary to language barriers, will prohibit the engagement and participation of patients in partnering to ensure adherence to required treatment plans and their overall health and wellness (Berkman et al., 2011, p. 8; Wilson-Stronks, Lee, Cordero, Kopp, & Galvez, 2008).

Health Literacy

Health literacy issues and ineffective communications place patients at greater risk of preventable adverse events. If a patient does not understand the implications of her or his diagnosis and the importance of prevention and treatment plans, or cannot access health care services because of communications problems, an untoward event may occur. The same is true if the treating physician does not understand the patient or the cultural context within which the patient receives critical information. Cultural, language, and communication barriers have great potential to lead to mutual misunderstandings between patients and their health care providers (The Joint Commission, 2007).

Health Literacy: Link to Patient Safety and an Expanded Scope in the Focus on Community Health and Wellness

As health care systems expand beyond acute care and hospitalization to focus on engaging patients in their health care and in promoting health and wellness to diverse populations and communities, cultural and language needs must be incorporated into the community health management strategies. In the pursuit of cultural and linguistic competence, health care systems must have a strategy to incorporate tenets of effective communication with a focus on health literacy. When literacy collides with health care, the issue of "health literacy"—defined as the degree to which individuals have the capacity to obtain, process, and understand basic health information and services needed to make appropriate health decisions—begins to cast a long patient-safety shadow (Nielsen-Bohlman, Panzer, Hamlin, & Kindig, 2004; The Joint Commission, 2007; USDHHS, Office of Disease Prevention and Health Promotion National Action Plan to Improve Health Literacy, 2010). As defined by Dr. Rudd, "Health Literacy happens when patients, or anyone on the receiving end of health communication, and providers, anyone on the giving end of health communication, truly understand one another" (Rudd, Anderson, Oppenheimer, & Nath, 2007, p. 176). Health literacy is critical to health care delivery, as the evidence strongly supports the fact that low health literacy is linked to higher risk of death and more ED visits and hospitalizations (Berkman et al., 2011, p. 8). Health literacy impacts health care outcomes as low literacy leads to less knowledge about illness and treatment, reduced use of preventive services, delayed access to care for several diseases, misuse of the ED, higher hospitalization rates, higher utilization and higher health care cost, and ultimately poor health outcomes (Berkman et al., 2011, p. 8). In a recent review of health literacy, Zarcadoolas and colleagues put forth an expanded and contemporary definition of health literacy whereby health literacy is presented as a dynamic process evolving over one's life being impacted by health status, demographic, sociopolitical, psychosocial, and cultural factors (Zarcadoolas, Pleasant, & Greer, 2005, p. 195). Zarcadoolas and colleagues define health literacy "as the wide range of skills and competencies that people develop to seek, comprehend, evaluate and use health information and concepts to make informed choices reduce health risks and increase quality of life" (Zarcadoolas et al., 2005, p. 195). This contemporary multidimensional model, which leads directly to an improvement of a population's health literacy, consist of the four domains as is illustrated in Figure 3.2.

1. Fundamental Literacy: Skills and strategies involved in reading, speaking, writing, and interpreting numbers

2. Science Literacy: The levels of competence with science and technology

3. Civic Literacy: Abilities that enable citizens to become aware of public issues and become involved in the decision-making process

4. Cultural Literacy: The ability to recognize and use collective beliefs, customs, world view, and social identity in order to interpret and act on health information (Zarcadoolas et al., 2005, p. 196).

This expanded model of health literacy is aligned with the findings of a 2006 Workshop on Improving Health Literacy hosted by the U.S. Surgeon General. This Surgeon General Workshop identified the public health consequences of limited health literacy, and reiterated the link between heath literacy

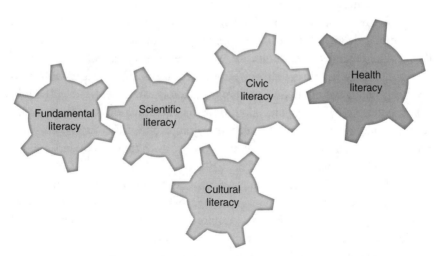

Figure 3.2 An expanded model of health literacy: Four central domains.

Adapted from Zarcadoolas, Pleasant, and Greer (2005).

and health outcomes. The workshop put forth limited health literacy as a major issue in public health society wide, and issued a nation-wide call to action to ensure that health information services meet the needs of the public (USDHHS, Office of Disease Prevention and Health Promotion National Action Plan to Improve Health Literacy, 2010).

Applications of the Expanded Model of Health Literacy to Individual Patient Care

MJ, the 72-year-old Haitian woman who presented to the ED with abdominal pain, and spoke French and Creole with very little understanding of English, interacted with a health care team whose main and only focus was on making a diagnosis so that life-saving treatment could be started. With regard to fundamental literacy (i.e., reading, writing, speaking, and numeracy), MJ had a fifth-grade French education. The medical team's descriptions of "diverticulitis" and surgery were described in a complex manner and were foreign to MJ, leading to increased anxiety and fear. The definition of diverticulitis and the surgical treatment strategy as presented by the medical team did not match the fundamental and science literacy of a population with a fifth-grade education. With regard to cultural literacy, the medical team initially did not recognize MJ's cultural beliefs and fears about illness and surgery, illustrating that cultural differences can lead to different interpretations and reactions to the same message.

The communication breakdown between MJ and her medical team resulted in a delay in diagnosis and treatment for diverticulitis and highlights the fact that "effective communication is a cornerstone of patient safety and that the safety of patients cannot be assured without mitigating the negative effects of low health literacy and ineffective communications on patient care" (The Joint Commission, 2007). The Joint Commission's accreditation standards underscore the fundamental right and need for patients to receive information—both orally and written—about their care in a way in which they can understand this information (The Joint Commission, 2010).

MJ's case facilitates an expanded view of health literacy whereby her health literacy is influenced by many components of her life including social, cultural, psychological, and economic components. A recent definition put forth by Sorenson and colleagues exemplifies this expanded dynamic scope of health literacy whereby "Health literacy is linked to literacy and entails people's knowledge, motivation and competences to access, understand, appraise, and apply health information in order to make judgments and take decisions in everyday life concerning health care, disease prevention and health promotion to maintain or improve quality of life during the life course" (Sorensen et al., 2012, p. 80).

Health Literacy Strategies for Health Care Organizations

Over 15 years of population health research underscore the fact that today's health information is presented in a way that is not comprehended by most Americans (USDHHS, Office of Disease Prevention and Health Promotion National Action Plan to Improve Health Literacy, 2010). The lack of clear health information and misunderstanding of the importance of prevention and self-management of chronic health conditions (e.g., diabetes mellitus, hypertension) eventually can lead to avoidance of necessary medical tests, lack of adherence to medication, and frequent ED visits (Nielsen-Bohlman et al., 2004). Recent research underscores the severity of limited health literacy in the United States as the most recent population data on literacy skills document no improvement in health literacy for the past decade with health literacy as a population health problem of great proportion affecting nearly 9 out of 10 English-speaking adults in the United States (Parker, 2008, pp. 1273–1276).

Publications by the IOM in 2004 and the Agency for Healthcare Research and Quality (AHRQ) in 2006 on the importance of health literacy to the health of the nation and the link with limited literacy on myriad health outcomes paved the way for major health professional organizations to develop and implement strategies to integrate tenets of health literacy in all aspects of the delivery of health care and the promotion of health and wellness to populations and communities (Nielsen-Bohlman et al., 2004; USDHHS, Office of Disease Prevention and Health Promotion National Action Plan to Improve Health Literacy, 2010).

The 2007 Joint Commission white paper titled *What Did the Doctor Say? Improving Health Literacy to Protect Patient Safety* provides compelling evidence linking effective communication to patient safety and issues a call to action and provides tactics for health care organizations to: (1) make effective communication an organization priority to protect the safety of patients; (2) meet the communication needs of patients across the continuum of care; and (3) focus and integrate policy changes that promote improved practitioner–patient communications (The Joint Commission, 2007).

In 2010, the USDHHS published the National Action Plan to Improve Health Literacy and presented limited health literacy as a public health problem. This document issued a call to action and provided seven goals and several strategies for medical societies, health care organizations, and medical and nursing schools to improve health literacy (USDHHS, Office of Disease Prevention and Health Promotion National Action Plan to Improve Health Literacy, 2010).

Two goals that are specifically pertinent to health care teams for the effective and safe delivery of patient and community centered care to diverse populations are:

1. Promote changes in the health care system that improve health information, communication, informed decision making, and access to health services

2. Increase basic research and the development, implementation, and evaluation of practices and interventions to improve health literacy

Research has documented the fact that several factors contribute to low health literacy. Factors adversely affecting health literacy include factors such as differences in language and cultural preferences, insufficient time and incentives for patient education, overuse of medical and technical terms to explain vital information, and lack of coordination among health care professionals (USDHHS, Office of Disease Prevention and Health Promotion National Action Plan to Improve Health Literacy, 2010). It is well documented that quality of clinician–patient communication is linked to patients' ability to follow instruction and affects health outcomes (Osborn, Paasche-Orlow, Davis, & Wolf, 2007, p. 376; Sudore et al., 2009, pp. 398–402; Williams, Davis, Parker, & Weiss, 2002, p. 383). Given the fact that few health care professionals have received formal education in communication and health literacy, there are now changes in educational and training curricula for medical professionals to integrate health literacy strategies and components into the delivery of care (Williams et al., 2002, p. 384; Yedidia et al., 2003, p. 1165).

Evolving knowledge suggests that changing the health care delivery system to address the factors that contribute to low health literacy may improve health care outcomes and the delivery of patient-centered care (Institute of Medicine, 2011). With regard to improving the health care delivery system to promote effective communication, informed decision making, and access to clinical services, the National Action Plan to Improve Health Literacy suggests 12 strategies for implementation by health care professionals, educators, health care executives, accreditation organizations and educators, and licensing and credentialing organizations. Educators, accreditation, licensing, and credentialing organizations are included as they play a critical role in shaping the training and practice standards for medical and public health professionals (USDHHS, Office of Disease Prevention and Health Promotion National Action Plan to Improve Health Literacy, 2010). The 12 strategies for all health care professionals, defined as anyone who is part of a health care or public health services team, are:

1. Use proven methods of checking patient understanding, such as the teach-back method, to ensure that patients understand health information and risk and benefit tradeoffs associated with treatment, procedures, tests, and medical devices

2. Use patient-centered technologies at all stages of the health care process to support information and decision-making needs of patients

3. Use direct and developmentally appropriate communication with children to build better understanding of their health and health care

4. Use different types of communication and tools with patients, including vetted pictures and models and scorecards, to support written and oral communication with patients and their caregivers

5. Use existing programs, such as AHRQ's "Questions Are the Answers," to prepare patients and providers for visits and structure their communication

6. Ensure that pharmacists provide the necessary counseling to consumers in language they understand for dispensed medications as required by law

7. Participate in ongoing training in health literacy, plain language, and culturally and linguistically appropriate service and encourage colleagues and staff to be trained

8. Advocate for a requirement in continuing education for health care providers who have been working in the field but have not participated in health literacy, cultural competency, and language access training

9. Create patient-friendly environments that facilitate communication by using architecture images and language to reflect the community and it values

10. Refer patients to adult education and English language programs

11. Refer patients to public and medical libraries to get more information and assistance with finding accurate and actionable health information

12. Use technology, including social media, to expand patients' access to the health care team and information (USDHHS, Office of Disease Prevention and Health Promotion National Action Plan to Improve Health Literacy, 2010)

The Affordable Care Act: A National Mandate for Health Equity to Ensure the Delivery of Quality Patient-Centered Care to Diverse Populations

Reforming the U.S. health care system was the top domestic priority of the 44th president of the United States when he was sworn into office in January 2009. Health Care reform was in critical need of improvement as racial/ethnic disparities in health and health care in the United States are persistent and well documented. Communities of color fare far worse than their White counterparts across a range of health indicators such as life expectancy, prevalence of chronic diseases, health status, and insurance coverage (Smedley et al., 2009).

In the last quarter of 2009, the U.S. House of Representatives and the U.S. Senate passed the Affordable Health Choices Act and the ACA. The ACA provides a comprehensive strategy to improve health and health services for racially and ethnically diverse populations. With its provisions to improve access, affordability, and quality of care the ACA lays a strong foundation for eliminating the legacy of health disparities (Andrulis, Siddiqui, Purtle, & Duchon, 2010).

The ACA includes several requirements that are unequivocally intended to reduce health disparities and improve the health of racially and ethnically diverse populations. Included among these provisions are two important strategies for the health care community: (1) focus on standardized data collection and reporting by race, ethnicity and language, and cultural competence education and training for health care professionals as an important strategy for improving the quality of care delivered to culturally and linguistically diverse populations, and (2) cultural competence training and education for health professionals as a credible strategy for improving the quality of care delivered to culturally and linguistically diverse patients. Additional provisions in the ACA with the power to reduce inequities in both health and health care, include an expansion of clinical and community-based prevention initiatives, funding for community health grants, and expanded health care access for underserved populations. Included in the ACA are new payment models that deviate from the fee-for service rates to a model that favor reimbursement for quality-driven, coordinated, population-based care. The new payment model in the ACA set into motion Medicare and Medicaid reimbursement and performance incentive plans for hospitals and physicians that could further help reduce health care inequities (Alberti, Bonham, & Kirch, 2013, p. 1620)

Health Literacy and the Affordable Care Act

Given the changing language and cultural demographics of the United States and the recent reports that about 87 million adults are considered functionally illiterate (Vernon, Trujillo, Rosenbaum, & DeBuono, 2007), the ACA, by extending health insurance coverage to close to 32 million lower-income adults, highlights the barriers faced by individual patients and therefore the critical need to incorporate health literacy into strategies for enrolling beneficiaries and delivering health care. National data suggest that only about 12% of adults have proficient health literacy (National Center for Education Statistics, U.S. Department of Education, 2010). Although low health literacy is prevalent across all demographic groups, it disproportionately affects non-White racial and ethnic groups, the elderly, individuals with lower socioeconomic status and education, people with physical and mental disabilities, those with limited English proficiency, and nonnative speakers of English (Nielsen-Bohlman et al., 2004). While the ACA does not focus clearly on health literacy, the success of the ACA arguably calls for a continued national focus on implementation of strategies to address low health literacy. Nearly 36% of America's adult population is considered functionally illiterate, with rates of low literacy found disproportionately among lower-income Americans eligible for publicly financed care through Medicaid (Somers & Mahadevan, 2010). Several provisions in the ACA with direct reference to health literacy are section 3501, which requires AHRQ researchers to be available to the public to reflect the varying needs of consumers and their diverse levels of health literacy, and section 5301, which has specific reference for training grants in cultural competence and health literacy (Somers & Mahadevan, 2010).

Given the fact that low health literacy is linked with poor health outcomes, medication errors, low rates of treatment compliance, and reduced use of preventive services and chronic disease management strategies, hospital readmission, and longer hospital stays, health literacy awareness and programs with targeted research and health literacy measurement metrics have been the focus of federal and state agencies as well as private health care organization and insurance companies (Somers & Mahadevan, 2010). Low health literacy has been estimated to cost the U.S. economy more than 100 billion dollars per year (Vernon et al., 2007).

Conclusion

As the population of the United States continues to become more diverse, there is a critical need for the integration of tenets of health literacy and cultural and linguistic competence into the paradigm for the delivery of health care for ethnically diverse populations. In diverse communities in the United States, health disparities are well documented. Integration of health literacy strategies and culturally and linguistically appropriate services in the health care delivery algorithm are essential for ensuring health equity. By customizing health care services to an individual's literacy level and culture and language preference, health care teams can ensure positive health outcomes for diverse populations. The delivery of health care services that are respectful of and responsive to the health beliefs, practices, and needs of diverse patients can ensure excellent health care outcomes in diverse communities.

References

Alberti, P. M., Bonham, A. C., & Kirch, D. G. (2013). Making equity a value in value-based health care. *Academic Medicine, 88*(11), 1619–1623.

Andrulis, D. P., Siddiqui, N. J., Purtle, J., & Duchon, L. (2010, July). *Patient Protection and Affordable Care Act of 2010: Advancing health equity for racially and ethnically diverse populations. The Joint Center.* Retrieved from http://www.jointcenter.org/research/patient-protection-and-affordable-care-act-of-2010-advancing-health-equity-for-racially-and

Benjamin, R. M. (2010). Surgeon general's perspective for improving health by improving health literacy. *Public Health Reports, 125*(6), 784–788.

Berkman, N. D., Sheridan, S. L., Donahue, K. E., Halpern, D. J., Viera, A., Crotty, K., . . . Viswanathan, M. (2011, March). *Health literacy interventions and outcomes: An updated systematic review. Evidence report/technology assessment no. 199.* Prepared by RTI International–University of North Carolina Evidence-based Practice Center under contract No. 290-2007-10056-I. AHRQ Publication No. 11-E006. Rockville, MD: Agency for Healthcare Research and Quality.

Betancourt, J. R., Green, A. R., & Carrillo, J. E. (2002). Cultural competence in health care: Emerging frameworks and practical approaches. *Commonwealth Fund, Quality of Care for Underserved Populations, 576.*

Betancourt, J. R., Renfrew, M. R., Green, A. R., Lopez, L., & Wasserman, M. (2012 September). *Improving patient safety systems for patients with limited English proficiency: A guide for hospitals.* AHRQ Publication No. 12-0041. Rockville, MD: Agency for Healthcare Research and Quality.

Colin, J. M., & Paperwall, G. (2003). People of Haitian heritage. In L.D. Purnell & B. J. Paulanka (Eds.), *Transcultural health care: A culturally competent approach* (2nd ed., pp. 517–543). Philadelphia, PA: F. A Davis.

Cooper University Health Care. (2013). Patient-family centered care. In *Patient guide.* Retrieved November 13, 2013, from http://www.cooperhealth.org/patient-guide/patient-family-centered-care

Cross, T., Bazmn, B. J., Dennis K. W., & Isaacs M. R. (1989). *Towards a culturally competent system of care* (Vol. 1). Washington, DC: CASSP Technical Assistance Center. Center for Child Health and Mental Health Policy, Georgetown University Child Development Center.

Frampton, S., Guastello, B., et al. (2008). *Patient centered care improvement guide.* Retrieved from Planetree (www.planetree.org) and Picker Institute (www.pickerinstitute.org)

Goode, T. D., Dunne, M. C., & Bronheim, S. M. (2006, October). *The evidence base for cultural and linguistic competency in health care.* New York, NY: The Commonwealth Fund.

Hasnain-Wynia R., & Wolf, M. S. (2010). Promoting health care equity: Is health literacy a missing link? *Health Services Research, 45,* 897–903.

Health Research & Educational Trust. (2011, July). *Institute for diversity in health management. building a culturally competent organization: The quest for equity in health care.* Chicago, IL: Author. Retrieved from www.hret.org/quality/projects/resources/cultural-competency_cp.pdf

Health Research & Educational Trust. (2013, August). *Reducing health care disparities: Collection and use of race, ethnicity and language data.* Chicago, IL: Author. Retrieved from www.hpoe.org

Institute of Medicine. (2001). *Crossing the quality chasm: A new health system for the 21st century.* Washington, DC: The National Academies Press.

Institute of Medicine. (2011). *Promoting health literacy to encourage prevention and wellness.* Workshop summary. Washington, DC: The National Academies Press.

National Center for Cultural Competence. (2010). *The compelling need for cultural and linguistic competence.* Retrieved November 13, 2013, from http://nccc.georgetown.edu /foundations/need.htm

Nielsen-Bohlman, L., Panzer, A., Hamlin, B., & Kindig, D. A. (Eds.). (2004). *Health literacy: A prescription to end confusion.* Washington, DC: The National Academies Press.

Osborn, C. Y., Paasche-Orlow, M. K., Davis, T. C., & Wolf, M. S. (2007). Health literacy: An overlooked factor in understanding HIV health disparities. *American Journal of Preventive Medicine, 33*(5), 374–378.

Pandya, C., Batalova, J., & McHugh, M. (2011). *Limited English proficient individuals in the United States: Number, share, growth, and linguistic diversity.* Washington, DC: Migration Policy Institute.

Parker, R. M. (2008). Preparing for an epidemic of limited health literacy: Weathering the perfect storm. *International Journal of General Medicine, 23*(8), 1273–1276.

Rudd, R. E., Anderson, J. E., Oppenheimer, S., & Nath, C. (2007). Health literacy: An update of public health and medical literature. In J. P. Comings, B. Garner, & C. Smith (Eds.), *Review of adult learning and literacy* (Vol. 7, pp. 175–204). Mahwah, NJ: Lawrence Erlbaum Associates.

Saha, S., Beach, M. C., & Cooper, L. A. (2008, November). Patient centeredness, cultural competence and healthcare quality. *Journal of the National Medical Association, 100*(11), 1275–1285.

Shrestha, L. B., & Heisler, E. J. (2011, March). *The changing demographic profile of the United States. Congressional Research Service.* Retrieved from http://www.fas.org/sgp/crs/misc/RL32701.pdf

Smedley, B. D., Stith, A. Y., & Nelson, A. R. (Eds.). (2009). *Unequal treatment: Confronting racial and ethnic disparities in health care* (with CD). Washington, DC: The National Academies Press.

Somers, S. A., & Mahadevan, R. (2010, November). *Health literacy implications of the Affordable Care Act.* Hamilton, NJ: Center for Health Care Strategies.

Sorensen, K., Van den Broucke, S., Fullam, J., Doyle, G., Pelikan, J., Slonska, Z., & Brand, H. (2012). Health literacy and public health: A systematic review and integration of definitions and models. *BMC Public Health,* 12, 80.

Sudore, R. L., Landefeld, C. S., Pérez-Stable, E. J., Bibbins-Domingo, K., Williams, B. A., & Schillinger, D. (2009). Unraveling the relationship between literacy, language proficiency, and patient-physician communication. *Patient Education and Counseling, 75*(3), 398–402.

The Joint Commission. (2007). *What did the doctor say? Improving health literacy to protect patient safety* (pp. 1–64). Oakbrook Terrace, IL: Author.

The Joint Commission. (2010). *Advancing effective communication, cultural competence, and patient- and family-centered care: A roadmap for hospitals.* Oakbrook Terrace, IL: Author.

U.S. Department of Education, Institute of Education Sciences, National Center for Education Statistics. (2010). *2003 National Assessment of Adult Literacy (NAAL).* Retrieved from http://nces.ed.gov/naal

U.S. Department of Health and Human Services, Office of Disease Prevention and Health Promotion. (2010). *National action plan to improve health literacy.* Washington, DC: Author.

U.S. Surgeon General & Department of Health and Human Services. (2007). *National standards on culturally and linguistically appropriate services.* Retrieved from http://minorityhealth.hhs.gov/templates/browse.aspx?lvl=2&lvlID=15

Ulmer, C., McFadden, B., & Nerenz, D.R. (2009). *Race, ethnicity, and language data: Standardization for health care quality improvement.* Washington, DC: National Academies Press.

Vernon, J., Trujillo, A. S., Rosenbaum, S., & DeBuono, B. (2007). *Low health literacy: Implications for national health policy.* George Washington University. Retrieved from http://sphhs.gwu.edu/departments/healthpolicy/CHPR/downloads/LowHealthLiteracyReport10_4_07.pdf

Williams, M. V., Davis, T., Parker, R. M., & Weiss, B. D. (2002). The role of health literacy in patient-physician communication. *Family Medicine, 34*(5), 383–389.

Wilson-Stronks, A., Lee, K. K., Cordero, C. L., Kopp, A. L., & Galvez, E. (2008). *One size does not fit all: Meeting the health care needs of diverse populations.* Oakbrook Terrace, IL: The Joint Commission.

Yedidia, M. J., Gillespie, C. C., Kachur, E., Schwartz, M. D., Ockene, J., Chepaitis, A. E., . . . Lipkin, M. Jr. (2003). Effect of communications training on medical student performance. *Journal of the American Medical Association, 290*(9), 1157–1165.

Zarcadoolas, C., Pleasant, A., & Greer, D. S. (2005). Understanding health literacy: An expanded model. *Health Promotion International, 20*(2), 195–203.

4

The Health Literacy Environment: Enhancing Access and Wayfinding

Terri Ann Parnell

M rs. Murphy, a 54-year-old executive assistant, had entered the hospital's main lobby and asked at the information desk where the preadmission testing area was? She had to have some tests done before her upcoming gynecological procedure. The lovely volunteer pointed and stated that she should "continue down this hall, when you get to the end make a left and follow it down until you see the sign for preadmission testing on your left."

Mrs. Murphy followed the instructions, but after the first left she forgot where to go next. She was not given any printed information to refer to nor was she able to scan the directions into her phone. She tried making eye contact with someone to ask again, but everyone was so busy as they hurried past her in the crowded hallway, and getting on and off the elevators. She kept walking trying to locate a sign for preadmission testing, while also looking for a friendly face to stop and ask for additional directions and clarification.

Finally, an employee stopped and asked if she needed assistance. He provided the additional information and off she went further down the long hallway. She turned where the employee explained to go and the large sign on the doorway simply said "PAT" in large, capital, red-colored, bold letters. She stood looking at the sign wondering if it was okay to enter. Finally she got the courage to open the door and cautiously entered. A nurse greeted her and asked if she could help her. Mrs. Murphy said, "I am here for preadmission testing, but the sign says this is where 'PAT' goes and my name is Mary Beth? Where should I go?"

Accessing and navigating throughout the health care system can be quite challenging and problematic to most consumers of health care. For the majority of persons going to a hospital, it is a time of stress, fear, and anticipation, which even under the best circumstances would make most encounters more difficult. Even if visiting someone for a happy occasion such as the birth of a new baby can bring anxiety and impact upon how one navigates throughout the facility. The health care built environment has been and continues to be confusing to most health facility users. Patients, caregivers, friends, and family experience unnecessary stress and confusion in these settings (Lee & Bauer, 2013).

Then imagine if you were you a limited English proficient (LEP) speaker, or from a totally different culture and you were trying to access or navigate through a health facility for the first time. Or you received instructions from your doctor's office to go to the imaging department for your procedure and you couldn't finds signs that referred to imaging because they all were labeled radiology or x-ray. Oftentimes, the words used in the hospital are not familiar to the layperson visiting. It can sometimes feel as if everyone had a special secret language.

There are many strategies that can assist health care facilities in enhancing patient's ability to initially find a facility and then navigate their way to their specific destination. External and internal signage, printed maps, and kiosks located in the lobby, are all tools that can enhance a person's ability to more easily move from one place to another. Sometimes too much complex medical terminology, organizational silos, and a haphazard pattern of expansion along with the predictable stress levels of patients and visitors make hospitals difficult to navigate (Cooper, 2010b). Although it is not very common to have nursing involved in signage and wayfinding planning, nurses are often the employees that are redirecting visitors or escorting them to their destination. They can be helpful in providing experiential information about the facility's current status as well as insight into what is and is not working well.

Access and Initial Entry Location

It can be quite difficult accessing a facility for the initial time, and especially so if the facility doesn't have visible signage on the exterior of the building. In addition, if there are several ways of arriving at the building, either by bus, train, or car, the facility may not have clearly visible and labeled signage at all multiple points of entry. Another aspect to keep in mind is the entranceway for the disabled. While a facility may provide special parking and transportation accommodations for the disabled, it should also incorporate the appropriate signage so that the patient or visitor feels safe and comfortable and also knows where to go during the transitional time from parking to the entrance of the building. A system that assists persons with the location of the entryway, adequate lighting, and maps with "you-are-here" locations clearly marked can assist in directing persons to their specific destination. The "you-are-here" map should be located so that it is viewable by all, preferably near an obvious landmark in the facility so that the orientation of the map is consistent with the reference points. If the orientation is not consistent with the facility, the signage can be more confusing than if it wasn't there.

In fact, signage is not always helpful and can in fact sometimes hinder a person's experience within health care facilities (Rousek & Hallbeck, 2011).

With over a million outpatient hospital visits a year (Hing, Hall, & Xu, 2008) and servicing an increasingly diverse patient population, it is vital that signage be understandable to all (Salmi, 2007). Signs will be more easily understood if they use everyday words or plain language and are consistent in their labeling. For example, label the outpatient area as "walk-in" rather than "ambulatory," or the cardiothoracic center as "cardiac center" or "heart center." Being consistent in your signage labeling is equally as important. The words or language used on signage is a major way a facility communicates with its customers (Carpman & Grant, 1993, p. 39). Upon making the complicated decisions for external signage, it is important to maintain consistency throughout the facility. Try to keep the nomenclature short and to the point, and use words that are understandable for the majority of your patient population.

In addition, outdoor areas near all entrances to the facility should have adequate waiting and seating areas. This is to accommodate persons waiting for cab rides or family members picking them up. Many facilities are now offering valet parking to their customers, which can provide an easier option for those parking a long distance away and walking to the main entrance. Valet parking also enhances the service experience for all.

The entrance way and main lobby can help in setting the tone for the facility. It provides a place to welcome your visitors. Signage can actually reach out and make your visitors feel more comfortable with their navigating experience

(Harkness, 2008). It is recommended that signage in the lobby of a facility have words of welcome and if possible an information desk with a sign explaining what it is (Rudd & Anderson, 2006). In fact, oftentimes, a person's first interaction with a hospital staff member is at the information desk in the main lobby or entry-way. In addition to providing an initial statement about the entire facility and welcoming the visitor, the entryway provides a transitional area where visitors can remove coats and begin to meet the staff, ask directions, and communicate and orient themselves for the first time (Carpman & Grant, 1993).

The skill set and training of the staff at the information desk staff is of critical importance as they can enhance the first impression of your facil-ity. Educating and training your front-line personnel at the information desk about speaking in plain language and being culturally sensitive can provide tremendous rewards. After all, they will be greeting visitors and outpatients, and providing directions on daily basis. If they are given the same educational opportunities as others in the organization, the communication culture will be more consistent throughout your facility.

Often, as a facility grows and expands it services, other entrances are added and the multiple "main entrances" can become confusing. How many times have you heard staff in your facility state to a patient being discharged to pick up the patient at the "old main entrance" or the "new main entrance." Additional signage, either free standing or mounted on the building should be added to clearly identify which entrance it is.

Staff must also try their best to refer to it as labeled. Sometimes when senior staff members are in the facility, they may refer to areas and buildings by the names they used to be years ago when they first began working. Over the years the building may have new donors and names may change, but the employee still refers to the building by its old name. An important and often overlooked area is assessing how staff members commonly refer to areas when giving visitors directions. Oftentimes, staff members can inadvertently further confuse the visitor as they may use a conflicting term or name.

The entryway signage should ideally include the facility's logo, the name of the entrance, hours of operation if applicable, as well as any immediate restric-tions or policies that all visitors must be aware of, such as no smoking (Cooper, 2010b). Upon entry into the facility a visitor should be able to then easily locate the directory.

Creating a Shame-Free, Welcoming Environment

All staff members can be of assistance in creating a shame-free environment. A shame-free environment is one that encourages individuals to ask for assistance when needed. Persons coming to an unfamiliar facility will feel welcome if there is staff available to greet them as they enter the lobby. These staff members can assist with the transition from the lobby to the person's specific destination. The staff member should ideally be in uniform and wear an identification badge that is easily visible. The clothing worn by employees in many health care facilities makes it difficult for visitors to know who they can reach out to and ask for assistance. A staff member in the lobby or at the main entrance in a distinguishable uniform and identification tag will assist in enhancing the environment and comfort level of the visitor.

An example that comes to mind of an environment that was not welcoming was when I once visited a hospital facility. Upon entering there was a desk off to side with staff that seemed to be volunteers and straight ahead was another rather tall desk with staff in security uniforms. It was a bit intimidating and not very friendly, as it appeared that the security presence was more important than the information desk. The employees in the security uniforms were the very first hospital employees I saw. Upon returning months later, the entire entranceway and lobby were redesigned. It was not only an esthetically pleasing but also warm and welcoming. Chairs and couches were added where visitors could stop and remove coats, or wait for other family members. The information desk remained to the left but it was clearly labeled and the staff were extremely attentive and friendly. They even added a kiosk next to it for those preferring to use the touch screen for directions. The biggest visual change was that the height of the desk immediately in front of the entrance way was lowered and redesigned. The security staff was still there but it was a more inviting environment. It no longer gave you the sense that you were walking into a police precinct. The redesign and openness of the area was much more inviting and welcoming. The lighting was changed, which provided a warm, more natural environment. The signage was also improved and the lobby was now an inviting and welcoming area where visitors could feel comfortable asking for directions and also a place to gather with their family members.

Health Care Wayfinding

Wayfinding is defined as "what people see, what they think about and what they do to find their way from one location to another" (Carpman & Grant, 1993, p. 66). Once a visitor is inside your facility, wayfinding assists the visitor with finding his or her way through the organization. Architects are very familiar with the term wayfinding although the reference to the term has been expanded a bit over the years. More recently, when speaking of wayfinding, the term now often infers the architecture and graphics, as well as the verbal and human interaction within the environment. When in a hospital setting, the human component of wayfinding is even more important (Passini & Arthur, 1992). Nursing can play a vital role in the wayfinding aspects involving human interaction within the environment.

The process of wayfinding is enhanced when a design solution provides aids to the intuitive navigational process. These clues may include maps or user guides, kiosks, written directions, or signage with lay terminology all with the intent of enhancing the users' ability to self-navigate throughout the facility (Cooper, 2010b).

Types of Wayfinding Information

Wayfinding information can be divided into three different types: appointments, personal interaction, and the environment (Murphy, 2012). Appointments can be made via many methods such as person-to-person phone calls, printed cards, and through electronics such as websites, e-mails, and texts. Each of these methods provides an opportunity to provide, reinforce, or clarify the directions and wayfinding information with the individual. Personal interaction is the most direct way to interact and provide information or directions to individuals (Murphy, 2012). It is also the most time consuming and often takes staff away from their scope of work to assist visitors. Both the exterior and interior environments can each provide orientation and direction cues that are extremely helpful to visitors as they make their way through a new facility. Although there are many ways to enhance the environment for wayfinding, signage remains the most universal way to communicate directions (Murphy, 2012).

Common Wayfinding Beliefs and Consequences

Oftentimes, wayfinding is done without much thought to the overall strategic plan. Commitment is needed from senior leadership down to every employee in the facility, as wayfinding is an ongoing initiative that will eventually impact upon every area, department, or subspecialty. When beginning the overall wayfinding plan, it is important to include education and training of employees. Training the staff to assist in enhancing the wayfinding program will provide the greatest impact as the program is rolled out and implemented and also as the hospital continues to expand and evolve (Cooper, 2010b, p. 13).

There are often many similar themes expressed by hospital leadership when discussing planning and allocating resources for a wayfinding plan. Below are several myths that can have a negative impact on the wayfinding plan and process (Cooper, 2010b, p. 12):

- Planning for an effective plan is a luxury.
- Preparing for the plan is a small commitment.
- Only large facilities need a formal wayfinding program.
- Forming an internal committee can fix the problem.
- Bigger and additional signs will fix the problem.
- Wayfinding is only about signage.
- It is a one-time investment and not an ongoing concern.
- Our program is too broken to fix.

Other common wayfinding beliefs are that "People will just ask for directions if they can't locate where they are going," or "Our hospital has been in this community for such a long time, everyone knows where to go or who to ask." These common beliefs can have a negative impact upon many areas.

Wayfinding is an often overlooked part of a hospital's ongoing strategic plan. Many issues have occurred in facilities due to a lack of planning over many years. These issues will not be corrected quickly, but rather require a staged ongoing plan and long-term commitment. Planning for an effective wayfinding program is vital to enhancing access and navigation, enhancing effective communication, as well as enhanced customer service.

The consequences to the above common beliefs can be costly in many areas. When a visitor or potential patient experiences frustration, it can directly relate to a decrease in customer experience and satisfaction. In addition, for persons having a difficult time finding where they are supposed to be going, a delay in arriving or a missed appointment can directly impact upon a loss in revenue. Another indirect impact can be the time invested by employees stopping what they are doing to provide directions or to escort visitors to their destination. Visitors may feel undue stress and anxiety as they are experiencing a feeling of confusion and disorientation. This stress and helplessness can exhibit itself in many ways, from anger and frustration, to panic in more extreme cases. When this occurs, the feelings are often turned toward the facility or hospital. Therefore, in a time when all facilities are trying their best to enhance the customer experience, an important area of focus and resources should be helping all persons find their destinations.

Signage

Let's read about a real-life wayfinding case scenario contributed by the hospital itself and reported by Cooper (2010a). The main campus of the Iowa Health System's signage had been neglected for many years. There was not a specific person responsible for signage, and therefore each department and area was posting its own. The only numbering system in place was for patient rooms. After many additions over many years, it was becoming more difficult to find one's way around the hospital. In fact, wayfinding was one of the top complaints on patient surveys. A wayfinding and signage study was done, and recommendations from a consulting firm were implemented. The reported enhanced results were immediate. The wayfinding complaints from patients and visitors dropped drastically, almost to zero. The hospital has since received many compliments on the effectiveness of the new signs and directories (Cooper, 2010a, p. 30).

The above scenario is just one example of how much the ease of navigation and the usability of the health care organization each depend upon the design and integration of proper signage. In fact, proper signage has a greater impact than simply providing directions. When designing the overall architecture of a building, planning for signage must be included as it has a significant impact on the wayfinding behavior of visitors (Rousek & Hallbeck, 2011).

Signage Color, Contrast, and Font Type

There has been much research done on the effects of signage design in different colors. Some colors provide contrast, while other colors may enhance a person's ability to notice the sign to begin with. When planning the color scheme for a hospital's wayfinding plan, one must also look to the codes and regulations as well as plan for flexibility for future growth and expansion. "In the United States, color-coding has been developed to lessen confusion and assist with decision making by using population stereotypes; warning labels are always displayed in red, caution information is always shown in yellow or amber and advisory information is shown in a color distinguishable from red and yellow" (Wickens, Lee, Liu, & Becker, 2004).

There are some color combinations that provide more contrast than others. One must consider the color contrast of the text and background upon the visibility, and whether the sign is an interior or exterior sign. Also keep in mind that persons who are color-blind will have difficulty interpreting signs that contain the colors red and green (Carpman & Grant, 1993).

The font type is also a consideration in the design phase of a wayfinding plan. Following all regulatory codes and standards is the most important priority and the first place to begin. If code dictates to use all capitals, of course they must be used. If all standards and codes reviewed do not dictate the type of lettering, then using mixed-case fonts can enhance the legibility of the signs. Use of upper and lower case, rather than all capital or upper case, has been shown to promote legibility as well as using serif fonts rather than sans serif fonts (Poncelet & Proctor, 1993; Strickland & Poe, 1989).

An article in *The New York Times* during the summer of 2012 indicated that "mixed-case signs are the wave of the future" (*The New York Times*, 2012). Although the New York City Department of Transportation does not have the same regulatory codes and standards as a health care facility, it is interesting to read that during their maintenance program, the city was beginning to replace older signs containing all uppercase lettering with new mixed-case lettering signs. Sign design nation-wide, governed by the *Manual on Uniform Traffic Control Devices*, states "the lettering for names of places, streets, and highways on conventional road guide signs shall be a combination of lowercase letters with initial upper case letters" (*Manual on Uniform Traffic Control Devices*, 2009, p. 138).

Terminology

Health care users need consistency and clarity in health care wayfinding (Richings, 2013). In addition to having the selected names used in a consistent manner across a health care facility, an often overlooked aspect that contributes to successful wayfinding is consistency of terms provided to the user in the previsit paperwork. If a patient receives instructions to report to the cardiac catheterization department for an angiogram but the signage uses the term Cath Lab, patients will have a difficult time finding the location. Or if the prescription received for blood tests states to go to the phlebotomy office on the first floor, and the actual area is labeled outpatient lab, it will be impossible to connect the two as being the same.

Another area of inconsistency with terminology is when the outpatient confuses the procedure they are having with the department or area they need to go to for the procedure. The outpatient may be looking for the x-ray department when he or she needs to go to the radiology department. Or perhaps the patient is looking for a sign indicating stress testing when he or she needs to find the cardiology department. Using terms and jargon that laypersons are not familiar with along with the inconsistency of terms used, creates an experience filled with confusion and stress.

Other Wayfinding Tools

A predominate visual component of most wayfinding programs is the signage. However, incorporating other interior and exterior components of the health facility into the wayfinding plan will assist in providing a more esthetically pleasing, robust, and comprehensive array of wayfinding tools.

Color Coding Buildings or Clinical Services

In addition to selecting colors for individual signs, some hospital facilities have selected colors for departments or buildings. For example, the pediatric area in the ambulatory clinics may be green allowing the person to look for the green area in the clinic building. Or a specific service line may be distinguished by colored flooring or walls painted in a specific color such as pink for the woman's wellness center. The use of accent lighting in a specific color can also visually guide visitors to their location.

Environmental Materials

In addition to signage, other exterior and interior materials can be used to contribute to a comprehensive wayfinding program. In the exterior environment, natural spaces, gardens, and specific architectural features can be utilized. The interior of the health facility can incorporate furnishings, lighting, statues, color, and other visual landmarks as communicative resources (Cooper, 2010b).

Successful wayfinding programs should incorporate both the external natural environment and architecture along with the interior built environment. It is truly a facility-wide priority, incorporating key facility stakeholders from across many disciplines, external experts in wayfinding design, the internal and external environments, a variety of communicative resources to meet the needs of a diverse population, and commitment from the facility to plan and educate all staff. The key to long-term success is the ability to be agile enough to change the wayfinding program as often as is needed in response to the changes occurring in the health care facility.

Regulations and Codes

This section is not intended to provide all the necessary regulatory codes and standards for one to follow, but rather to provide an overview of the importance of standards, regulations, and concepts that should be discussed with those that have an expertise in this area. Whenever developing health care signage for what is considered public places, such as hospitals and health care facilities, there are a variety of federal, state, and local building codes and standards. The most important of these regulations is the Americans with Disabilities Act (ADA). The ADA is civil rights legislation developed by the Department of Justice and administered by individual states (Hablamos Juntos, 2010b). Within the ADA, there is a section that specifically relates to signage (Rousek & Hallbeck, 2011). This section provides guidelines on the width, height, width-to-height ratio, character and number height, size, character case, font, raised character height, finish material, and background contrast, as well as mounting location of the signs used within a facility (Rousek & Hallbeck, 2011). It is further divided into interior and exterior signage. The ADA also sets the standards for tactile signage. It has been "recognized that signs needed for the blind and the visually impaired require two different types of sign: small sans serif tactile letters for the blind and larger letters with greater color contrast for the visually impaired" (Cooper, 2010b).

The Joint Commission standards do not specifically address signage and wayfinding standards; however, it has suggested recommendations such as translating signage into the top languages encountered by the organization (Cooper, 2010b, p. 95). The National Standards for Culturally and Linguistically Appropriate Services in Health Care also refers to having signage available in the languages of the patients served.

In an effort to assist in communicating to an increasingly diverse patient population, facilities are utilizing universal symbols that may be better understood by all who frequent the hospital. Some suggested universal symbols are those developed by Hablamos Juntos Language Policy and Practice in Healthcare (Cooper, 2010b).

In addition, there are standards and codes that apply to safety that set the expectation for areas such as fire safety and evacuation, elevators, stairwells, biohazards, and the laboratory. Look around the next time you are in a hospital or health care organization and you will also see signage for communications such as visiting-hour policies, smoking policies, handwashing, Health Insurance Portability and Accountability Act (HIPAA), or cell phone use. To complicate the regulatory aspect of signage even further, the standards, codes, or regulations are often being updated or new expectations are created. In addition, there are often different regulatory expectations for ambulatory care facilities, extended care facilities, or medical office buildings (Cooper, 2010b). The regulatory component of signage is a vital aspect of the plan and these items must be incorporated into the visual design phase for wayfinding in a health care facility.

Health care facilities need to address the demand for the increasing growth of LEP persons entering their facilities. Experts in design and wayfinding are establishing best practices that will assist persons with limited literacy and with LEP to more easily access and navigate health care services. Although regulatory expectations should be incorporated into the preliminary overall design plan, it can be rather overwhelming for health care executives to locate and interpret the appropriate codes for their facility; therefore it is best to consult with the experts early on in the planning phase.

Limited English Proficient Persons

When an individual speaks a language other than English, signage recognition becomes more difficult. The lack of language skills creates health risks for that

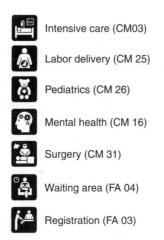

Figure 4.1 Selected Hablamos Juntos universal symbols © 2010.
Source: Hablamos Juntos (2010a).

patient population and adds an additional burden to the health care system (Cowgill & Bolek, 2003). One way to enhance communication with a diverse population is through the use of universal symbols in signage that can be collectively understood by all.

Hablamos Juntos means "we speak together," and is a program funded by The Robert Wood Johnson Foundation to improve patient–provider communication for Latinos. Hablamos Juntos, through an initiative called Signs That Work (STW), studied the communicative potential of graphic symbols and tested these symbols in regard to wayfinding for diverse limited English-speaking visitors to health care facilities (Hablamos Juntos, 2010a). A total of 54 symbols are now available in the public domain. The symbols are divided into three categories: administrative, facility, or imaging services, with the majority of symbols in the clinical or medical services category. The use of universal symbols can help to make all visitors more comfortable and confident as they navigate through unfamiliar health care facilities (Figure 4.1).

Universal symbols can enhance the effectiveness and efficiency in helping all persons navigate through complex health care facilities. They can be easier for patients to see and understand and are flexible, simple to implement, and can be integrated into other complex sign, print, and Internet strategies (Hablamos Juntos, 2010b).

Elderly

In a reported study of older adults and the emergency department, the environment of an emergency department was assessed to measure the impact upon the care of older adults aged 75 and over. Results indicated "orientation and way-finding cues, and access to the emergency department (parking, bus stop) and amenities (bathrooms, walkways and distance to other areas) presented challenges" (Kelley, Parke, Jokinen, Stones, & Renaud, 2011, p. 8). Recommendations to the physical environment included the enhancement of wayfinding including orientation and signage. Incorporating into wayfinding were the use of languages, symbols, graphics, and clocks as suggested ways to enhance wayfinding for the older adult. For the elderly population, problems with spatial orientation can also have a long-term impact and may even affect an older person's sense of control (Carpman & Grant, 1993). The use of technology is often perceived as an enemy by older populations, and especially those who have visual impairments (Lee & Bauer, 2013).

Pediatrics

Several studies have shown that there are distinct differences in the way younger and older children navigate through hospital settings. In addition "department names that were easier to pronounce, remember and understand and which related to departmental cues were easier to remember for both children and adults" (Pham, 2012). The trend of building hospital atria began in the 1960s to provide a very distinct and visible entrance along with easier point of reference and movement. The atrium model eventually began to be incorporated into pediatric hospitals. Although the reason for this is not clear, it is felt that creating a mall-like setting helps to provide an environment that is similar to a fun public space for children (Adams, Theodore, Goldenberg, McLaren, & McKeever, 2010). Hospital wayfinding for children often focuses on familiar themes such as nature or seasons. It is incorporated to help compartmentalize and divide areas and departments within the hospital. The inclusion of colorful art, mobiles, murals, and paintings helps create and support an environment of healing and also offer opportunities to provide playful distractions. Younger children are more sensitive to the changes appreciated in their environment and often quickly notice a change in colors on the walls or floor tiles, while older children have the ability to identify and use landmarks and are quickly able to infer shortcuts and develop cognitive maps (Pham, 2012). Although many agree that children should participate in the planning and evaluation of a hospital's nonmedical space, additional research is needed to determine effect of design on well-being (Adams et al., 2010).

Summary

Collaborating with a thoughtfully selected internal facility committee and a wayfinding design expert, and executing an initial needs assessment are the preliminary steps in planning a wayfinding project. Collectively, it is important to then determine the project goals, timelines, measurement criteria, branding design, and budget. Enhancing the health literacy environment for all users is more than just placing new signs around the facility. It incorporates branding, product positioning, code compliance, and utilitarian communications (Cooper, 2010b, p. 57). Wayfinding significantly impacts patient-centered care and patient satisfaction and can also assist in improving the bottom line (Lee & Bauer, 2013). Nurses can contribute as patient advocates as they are keenly aware of how their patients, families, and visitors access, navigate, and experience the overall facility. Ultimately, wayfinding is a direct extension of a health care facility's branding statement (Lee & Bauer, 2013).

References

Adams, A., Theodore, D., Goldenberg, E., McLaren, C., & McKeever, P. (2010). Kids in the atrium: Comparing architectural intentions and children's experiences in a pediatric hospital lobby. *Social Science and Medicine, 70,* 658–667.

Carpman, J. R., & Grant, M. A. (1993). *Design that cares. Planning health facilities for patients and visitors* (2nd ed.). San Francisco, CA: Jossey-Bass.

Cooper, R. (2010a). *Successful signage. How hospitals have solved wayfinding challenges.* Retrieved from http://www hfmmagazine.com

Cooper, R. (2010b). *Wayfinding for healthcare. Best practices for today's facilities.* Chicago, IL: Health Forum Inc, American Hospital Association Company.

Cowgill, J., & Bolek, J. (2003). *Symbol usage in health care settings for people with limited English proficiency: Part one, evaluation of use of symbol graphics in medical settings.* Scottsdale, AZ: JRC Design.

Dunlap, D. (2012). Like spelling, capitalization now counts on street signs. *New York Times.* Retrieved from http://cityroom.blogs.nytimes.com/2012/08/14/throughout-the-city-a-new-generation-of-street-signs/?_r=0

Hablamos Juntos. (2010a). *Universal symbols in health care: Tools for the development of a symbols-based wayfinding system.* Retrieved from http://www.hablamosjuntos.org/signage/symbols/default.using_symbols.asp

Hablamos Juntos. (2010b). *Universal symbols in health care workbook. Executive summary. Best practices for sign systems.* Retrieved from http://www.hablam osjuntos.org/signage/symbols/default.using_symbols.asp

Harkness, L. (2008, December 20). What exactly is "wayfinding"? *Main Street News,* No. 235.

Hing, E., Hall, M. J., & Xu, J. (2008). National Hospital Ambulatory Medical Care Survey: 2006 Outpatient Department summary. U.S. Department of Health and Human Services. *National Health Statistics Report,* No. 4.

Kelley, M. L., Parke, B., Jokinen, N., Stones, M., & Renaud, D. (2011). Senior-friendly emergency department care: An environmental assessment. *Journal of Health Services Research and Policy, 16*(1), 6–12.

Lee, D., & Bauer, C. (2013). *Wayfinding elements in the environment of care. Health facilities management.* Retrieved from http://www.hfmmagazine.com/hfmmagazine/jsp/articledisplay.jsp?dcrpath=HFMMAGAZINE/Article/data/04APR2013/0413HFM_FEA_interiors&domain=HFMMAGAZINE

Manual on Uniform Traffic Control Devices (MUTCD). (2009). *U.S. Department of Transportation, Federal Highway Administration.* Including Revision 1 and 2, May 2012. Retrieved from http://mutcd.fhwa.dot.gov/pdfs/2009r1r2/pdf_index.htm

Murphy, P. (2012). *Wayfinding planning for healthcare facilities.* White Paper. Lafayette, CA: GNU Group.

Passini, R., & Arthur, P. (1992). *Wayfinding: People, signs and architecture* (1st ed.). New York, NY: McGraw-Hill.

Pham, L. T. (2012). *Q & A: Finn Butler on wayfinding design.* SmartPlanet blog. Retrieved from http://www.smartplanet.com/blog/global-observer/q-a-finn-butler-on-wayfinding-design/5234

Poncelet, G. M., & Proctor, L. F. (1993). Design and development factors in the production of hypermedia based courseware. *Canadian Journal of Educational Communication, 22*(2), 91–111.

Richings, A. (2013). *Healthcare wayfinding: That name makes me sick!* Retrieved from http://www.endpoint.co.uk/healthcare-wayfinding-that-name-makes-me-sick

Rousek, J. B., & Hallbeck, M. S. (2011). Improving and analyzing signage within a healthcare setting. *Applied Ergonomics, 42,* 771–784.

Rudd, R. E., & Anderson, J. E. (2006). *The health literacy environment of hospitals and health centers: Partners for action; making your healthcare facility literacy-friendly.* Boston, MA: The National Center for the Study of Adult Learning and Literacy, (U.S.) Institute of Education Sciences.

Salmi, P. (2007). Wayfinding design: Hidden barriers to universal access. *Implications, 5*(8), 1–6.

Strickland, R. M., & Poe, S. E. (1989). Developing a CAI graphic simulation model guidelines. *The Journal of Technological Horizon in Education, 16*(7), 88–92.

Wickens, C. D., Lee, J. D., Liu, Y., & Becker, S. E. (2004). *An introduction to human factors engineering.* Upper Saddle River, NJ: Prentice Hall.

The Health Literacy Tipping Point

Terri Ann Parnell

Health literacy is relevant across an individual's life span and at every point across the health care continuum. Unlike the earlier research on health literacy that focused primarily on an individual's deficits or how to measure a person's health literacy level, there is now more of a focus on building patient–provider partnerships and attempting to minimize the gap between an individual's health literacy skills and the skills and demands of providers and health care systems.

Over the past few decades, leaders from the federal government, scientists, health researchers, health policy experts, and health professionals have together attempted to address the evolving concept of health literacy. They have raised awareness regarding the magnitude of the issue and implications of low health literacy, and have participated in multiple research papers, reports, plans, and workshops to share evidence-based strategies that address low health literacy in our communities and the populations served. These activities and publications help to provide the foundation necessary to promote the health literacy agenda and truly integrate health literacy into providing quality patient-centered care.

Healthy People 2010 was released by the U.S. Department of Health and Human Services [USDHHS] in January 2000 as a comprehensive health promotion and disease prevention agenda. The two overarching goals that guided the objectives developed were to increase quality and years of healthy life and to eliminate health disparities (USDHHS, 2000a). These national goals and

objectives were designed to help guide health promotion and disease prevention efforts in the United States to improve the health of all people. The specific goal of using communication strategically to improve health is within the
health communication chapter and contains objectives that monitor availability
of Internet access, health-related websites, and health literacy. This helped to
identify health literacy as a public health concern and also assisted in setting
objectives on a national level.

In the landmark publication, *Health Literacy: A Prescription to End
Confusion* (2004), health literacy was further defined; origins, consequences, and
possible solutions were described; and conceptual frameworks were provided.
One framework helped to identify health literacy as the "bridge between literacy skills and abilities of the person and the health context" (Nielsen-Bohlman,
Panzer, & Kindig, 2004, p. 32). The second framework assisted with providing a
visual to help identify the sectors that should be responsible for health literacy
and possible interventions. This report called upon the collaboration of educators, health professionals, researchers, government, and the community to
implement strategies to enhance health literacy. *Health Literacy: A Prescription
to End Confusion* called upon enhanced education in health literacy for all professional curricula in health and health-related fields such as medicine, nursing,
pharmacy, public health social work, and dentistry. In addition, it recommended
continuing education and clinical practice experiences to enhance health literacy for health professionals and health care staff. Health literacy was reported
as a critical component to the health of all individuals and the nation.

The U.S. Department of Education (2003) completed the National
Assessment of Adult Literacy (NAAL), the first national assessment in the
United States to measure health literacy. It assisted in establishing a founda-
tional baseline for future measurement of health literacy. (See Chapter 1, "What
Is Health Literacy?")

The USDHHS formed a Health Literacy Workgroup in 2004 under the
guidance of the Office of Disease Prevention and Health Promotion. The workgroup's commitment was to improve the health literacy of all Americans and
fostered collaboration among many agencies to raise awareness of the magnitude of the issue. In 2006, the workgroup members formed a steering committee and spearheaded the Surgeon General's Workshop on Improving Health
Literacy. The goal of this inaugural workshop was to present "the state of the
science in the field of health literacy from a variety of perspectives, including
those of health care organizations and providers, the research community, and
educators" (Office of the Surgeon General, 2006). After the 1-day workshop,

one conclusion was that the context of health literacy is not an individual shortfall but must be looked at across larger systems including social, cultural, educational, and public health systems. The workgroup also concluded that in order to expect consumers of health care to follow instructions and change their behaviors, all health professionals must provide clear and understandable health information. Additionally, we cannot advance in the fields of medical research and health information technology without addressing health literacy. Finally, although it has been demonstrated that we have enough information to begin to enhance health literacy, there is certainly a need for more research.

The inception of the Institute of Medicine (IOM) Roundtable on Health Literacy began in 2006. The Roundtable was convened to bring together leaders with an interest and role in enhancing health literacy from academia, industry, government, foundations, and associations as well as patient and consumer interests (IOM, 2006). It has developed work groups and activities focused on health insurance reform, oral health literacy, international health literacy, and the development of attributes for a health literate organization. The Roundtable on Health Literacy provides a stimulating forum for discussion and sharing of knowledge, expertise, and best practice across many companies, disciplines, and groups in both private and public sectors.

The Joint Commission (2007) report *"What Did the Doctor Say?"*: *Improving Health Literacy to Protect Patient Safety* was a call to action for all those who influence, develop, or deliver safe, high-quality health care. This report highlighted the communication gaps that exist between the abilities and skills of the persons receiving health care and the professionals providing health care. Research has well demonstrated that the information and materials provided to persons receiving care far exceed the individual's ability and skills necessary to understand and act upon this information.

The Joint Commission's accreditation standards stress that all patients have the right to receive information in a way they can understand. This applies to all information, whether it is written or orally communicated. "Effective communication is a cornerstone for patient safety" (The Joint Commission, 2007, p. 5). Nurses play a vital role and have a responsibility to present the information in a health literate way and be 50/50 partners in this communication relationship. It is vital to patient safety and patient outcomes.

"What Did the Doctor Say?" was an instrumental report focusing on the negative effect that low health literacy and ineffective communication have upon patient care (The Joint Commission, 2007). The report suggested several recommendations that, if followed, would help decrease communication-related

errors, help enhance health literacy, and help enhance the patient–provider relationship. One recommendation is to make communication an organizational priority to help enhance patient safety. In doing so, it is important for health care organizations to be familiar with the communities they serve. Although health literacy is a cross cutting priority and we should use a "universal precautions" approach, being aware of the organization's demographics will be of assistance in identifying communities that may have lower educational levels or lower socioeconomic status, which are potential contributing factors to low health literacy. Raising staff awareness regarding low health literacy and providing health literacy education and training to all staff will assist in enhancing patient safety. Providing patient resources for language and communication access services and creating an organizational culture of patient centeredness, patient safety, and patient satisfaction are all steps toward making patient safety an organizational priority.

A second recommendation from the report is to address all patient's communication needs across the continuum of care. This sounds like a simple task; however, a patient's health literacy skills are not always easily identified. Persons with low health literacy often have developed an amazing ability to adapt to situations. As nurses we must use a "universal precaution" approach as we do with handwashing for prevention of infection. We don't wash our hands only for patients we think may more easily become infected; we wash our hands at each and every patient encounter, each and every time. Health literacy should be an "always event" just like handwashing. A focus on access and entry into all points of care, transitions of care and hand-off communication, medication reconciliation, and self-management of disease will assist in enhancing patient safety.

Enhancing patient safety requires time to assess each patient's needs, provide individualized patient education in plain language, and incorporate teach-back to ascertain that your patient understands what was taught. Currently, the health care system does not look upon this valuable encounter as a reimbursable event. Therefore, the third recommendation is to pursue policy changes that help to promote and enhance patient–provider communications. The health care system needs to foster a culture of patient centeredness and allow and reimburse providers to spend more time with patients for education and effective communication.

On October 13, President Obama signed into law the "Plain Writing Act of 2010." The purpose of this Act is to "improve the effectiveness and accountability of Federal agencies to the public by promoting clear government communication that the public can understand and use" (The Plain Writing

Act, 2010). Under this Act, the responsibilities of each federal agency include the designation of one or more senior officials for oversight of the implementation of this Act, communicate the requirements of and train agency employees in plain writing, appoint a contact to receive and respond to public input, establish a process for ongoing compliance, and create a sustainable plain-writing section of the agency's website accessible from the home page. The agencies must use plain language in documents that are necessary for receiving federal government benefit or service or filing taxes, and, in addition, any documents that provide information about federal government benefits and services or documents that explain to the public how to comply with any federal government requirements. One example of improvements made by the Food and Drug Administration because of this Act is the over-the-counter drug label format (Figures 5.1 and 5.2). This illustrates an example of using visual explanations to show information in a clear and understandable way.

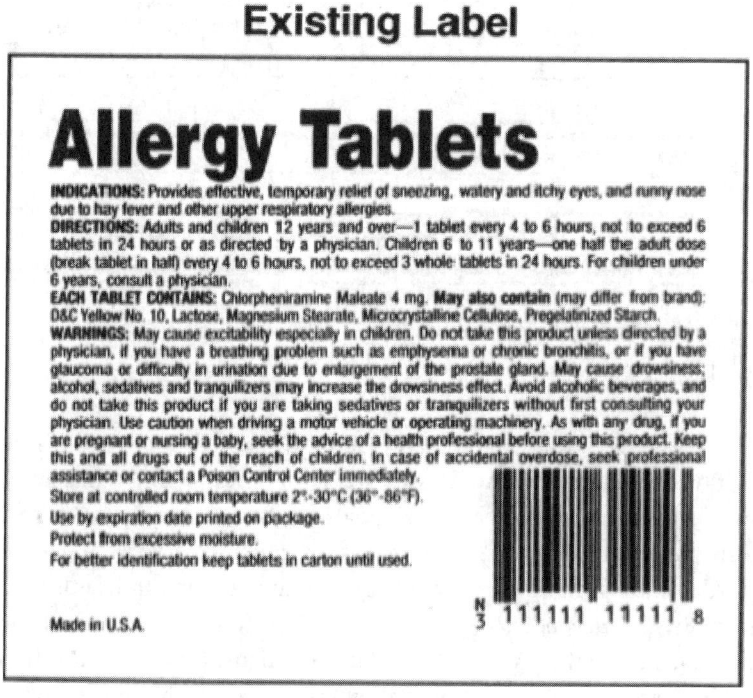
Existing Label

Allergy Tablets

INDICATIONS: Provides effective, temporary relief of sneezing, watery and itchy eyes, and runny nose due to hay fever and other upper respiratory allergies.
DIRECTIONS: Adults and children 12 years and over—1 tablet every 4 to 6 hours, not to exceed 6 tablets in 24 hours or as directed by a physician. Children 6 to 11 years—one half the adult dose (break tablet in half) every 4 to 6 hours, not to exceed 3 whole tablets in 24 hours. For children under 6 years, consult a physician.
EACH TABLET CONTAINS: Chlorpheniramine Maleate 4 mg. **May also contain** (may differ from brand): D&C Yellow No. 10, Lactose, Magnesium Stearate, Microcrystalline Cellulose, Pregelatinized Starch.
WARNINGS: May cause excitability especially in children. Do not take this product unless directed by a physician, if you have a breathing problem such as emphysema or chronic bronchitis, or if you have glaucoma or difficulty in urination due to enlargement of the prostate gland. May cause drowsiness; alcohol, sedatives and tranquilizers may increase the drowsiness effect. Avoid alcoholic beverages, and do not take this product if you are taking sedatives or tranquilizers without first consulting your physician. Use caution when driving a motor vehicle or operating machinery. As with any drug, if you are pregnant or nursing a baby, seek the advice of a health professional before using this product. Keep this and all drugs out of the reach of children. In case of accidental overdose, seek professional assistance or contact a Poison Control Center immediately.
Store at controlled room temperature 2°-30°C (36°-86°F).
Use by expiration date printed on package.
Protect from excessive moisture.
For better identification keep tablets in carton until used.

Made in U.S.A.

N 3 111111 11111 8

Figure 5.1 Over-the-counter drug label—Before.

Source: The Plain Language Writing Act (2010).

New Standard Labeling Format

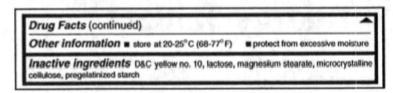

Drug Facts

Active ingredient (in each tablet)	Purpose
Chlorpheniramine maleate 2 mg..	Antihistamine

Uses temporarily relieves these symptoms due to hay fever or other upper respiratory allergies: ■ sneezing   ■ runny nose   ■ itchy, watery eyes   ■ itchy throat

Warnings

Ask a doctor before use if you have
■ glaucoma   ■ a breathing problem such as emphysema or chronic bronchitis
■ trouble urinating due to an enlarged prostate gland

Ask a doctor or pharmacist before use if you are taking tranquilizers or sedatives

When using this product
■ drowsiness may occur   ■ avoid alcoholic drinks
■ alcohol, sedatives, and tranquilizers may increase drowsiness
■ be careful when driving a motor vehicle or operating machinery
■ excitability may occur, especially in children

If pregnant or breast-feeding, ask a health professional before use.
Keep out of reach of children. In case of overdose, get medical help or contact a Poison Control Center right away.

Directions

adults and children 12 years and over	take 2 tablets every 4 to 6 hours; not more than 12 tablets in 24 hours
children 6 years to under 12 years	take 1 tablet every 4 to 6 hours; not more than 6 tablets in 24 hours
children under 6 years	ask a doctor ▼

Drug Facts (continued)   ▲

Other information ■ store at 20-25°C (68-77°F)   ■ protect from excessive moisture

Inactive Ingredients D&C yellow no. 10, lactose, magnesium stearate, microcrystalline cellulose, pregelatinized starch

Figure 5.2   Over-the-counter drug label—After.

Source: The Plain Language Writing Act (2010).

In early 2010, the United States Congress passed the Patient Protection and Affordable Care Act (ACA), as part of Congress's comprehensive health reform legislation. The law's primary goals are to increase access to coverage, regulate the private insurance industry to allow more Americans into the system at affordable rates, and begin to control the rate of growth in health care costs (Somers & Mahadevan, 2010, p. 7). To assist in meeting these goals, efforts are needed to enhance the provision of culturally, linguistically, and health-literate care. There are many provisions throughout the ACA that either directly or indirectly recognize the need for enhanced health literacy of the populations served. Although health literacy is not a main theme, it is difficult to imagine how health care reform can be successful without increasing our health literacy efforts at a national level. Health literacy–specific opportunities exist in six of the health and health care domains in the legislation, including coverage expansion, equity, workforce, patient information, public health and wellness, and quality improvement (Somers & Mahadevan, 2010, p. 4). Health literacy opportunities within these domains include the enrollment of expanded populations in 2014, having patient information and patient education that meets the needs of the populations being served, creating efficient health care delivery models that assist with chronic disease management and self-management of illness, and ensuring equitable care for all populations. In addition, the law includes the ability to communicate health information clearly so that it is understood, culturally appropriate, and patient centered. Persons with low health literacy will have more difficulty benefiting from the ACA. Low health literacy is more prevalent among lower-income Americans eligible for publicly financed care through Medicaid or Medicare (Kutner, Greenberg, & Baer, 2006). With the implementation of the ACA, the breadth and scope of persons newly eligible are likely to increase. Nurses and advanced practice nurses will play a vital role in providing care under the ACA and have a tremendous opportunity to assist in the efforts to make these opportunities clear and understandable to all.

The *National Action Plan (NAP) to Improve Health Literacy* was released in May 2010 in an effort to engage multiple stakeholders in a similar vision to improve health literacy and create a health literate society. The NAP is based on two principles—the first being that everyone has the right to health information that helps them make informed decisions, and, second, that all health services should be delivered in a way that is understandable and beneficial to health, longevity, and quality of life (USDHHS, 2010). It is the responsibility of health professionals to communicate in an understandable way. Without effective communication, we cannot expect consumers of health care to change behaviors and adapt to a healthy lifestyle. The overarching vision informing the NAP is that of a society that provides everyone with access to accurate and actionable health information, delivers person-centered health information and services, and supports lifelong learning and skills to promote good health (USDHHS, 2010, p. 1). The NAP describes seven goals that emphasize the importance of improving health literacy and strategies to achieve them. The Plan was a collaborative effort of many individuals, public and private stakeholder organizations, and town hall partners. It will take the combined efforts of all organizations and individuals collaborating in a coordinated fashion to improve the accessibility, usability, understandability, quality, and safety of health care. The NAP has provided the overarching goals and identified the strategic priorities needed to pursue a health literate society. Eliminating barriers and enhancing the way health care and health professionals, educators, and the media communicate health information offer the best way to achieve a society that is health literate (USDHHS, 2010, p. 6).

In 2010, The Joint Commission published a monograph entitled, *Advancing Effective Communication, Cultural Competence and Patient and Family Centered Care: A Roadmap for Hospitals*. This was an effort to assist hospitals in identifying and addressing the nonclinical areas of health care that are essential components of providing quality and safe patient care. Effective communication, cultural competence, and patient- and family-centered care are no longer perceived as just a patient's right. Research has demonstrated that providing patient-centered care incorporating effective communication and cultural competence can positively impact patient satisfaction and also adherence to prescribed treatment (Wolf, Lehman, Quinlin, Zullo, & Hoffman, 2008). *A Roadmap for Hospitals* provides methods for hospitals to improve upon their efforts to ensure that all patients, regardless of language, communication, mobility needs, culture, health literacy level, or sexual identity, receive the same safe and quality care. The format of *Roadmap for Hospitals* follows the main areas a patient may encounter along the continuum of care from admission and assessment, to treatment, discharge, or transfer and end-of-life care. The *Roadmap* is not prescriptive in its recommendations but rather makes broad suggestions with practice examples. It provides a comprehensive way that hospitals can support effective communication, cultural competence, and patient- and family-centered care.

While The Joint Commission's *Roadmap* was a resource specifically for hospitals, the *Health Literacy Universal Precautions Toolkit* (Agency for Healthcare Research and Quality [AHRQ], 2010) was developed specifically to be used by all staff in an adult or pediatric primary care practice setting. The University of North Carolina at Chapel Hill tested the toolkit at the request of the AHRQ. "Universal precautions" is when we perform certain activities to minimize risk for everyone, even though it is not always clear which patient it may effect. For example, in the hospital or health care setting, handwashing, the use of gloves, and aseptic technique are all examples of universal precautions. We perform these activities with all patients to minimize risk. The *Health Literacy Universal Precautions Toolkit* offers to minimize the risk that a consumer of health care will not understand the health or medication information or discharge instructions he or she is given. Health care professionals are not always aware which of their patients may have low health literacy skills. Even well-educated individuals can have low health literacy at certain health care encounters. They may have been educated, hold a job, be well spoken, and appear to function very well. The toolkit suggests that everyone may have low health literacy at times and have difficulty understanding health information. Creating an environment where we have practices in place to promote a shame-free environment will promote understanding for all patients, not just the patients you may think have low health literacy. It incorporates tools to enhance oral and written communication and tools that improve self-management and empowerment. The toolkit promotes a team approach that will assist with positive changes in the practice setting for patients of all literacy levels.

In December 2010, the USDHHS released Healthy People 2020, the revised 10-year goals and objectives for health promotion and disease prevention for the nation (USDHHS, 2000b). Everyone has the potential ability to prevent disease and manage wellness; however, there continues to be a mismatch between the increasing complex demands of the health care system and the skill set of individuals accessing this care. When disparities exist in access to health services, the implications can be less use of preventive care, higher hospital admissions, and poor health outcomes (Berkman et al., 2004). The goals and objectives of Healthy People 2020 present an opportunity to help prevent avoidable disease.

There are many objectives related to health literacy in the Health Communication and Health Information Technology topic area. Several objective examples are to improve the health literacy of the population, increase the percentages of people who state their health care professionals have adequate communication skills, are involved in decisions about their health, and use electronic personal health records. This topic area also incorporates health care professionals providing treatment instructions to care for a health condition or illness, offering to help with the completion of forms, and asking patients to describe how they will follow through with the instructions provided. Utilizing Healthy People 2020 as the roadmap to monitor and report progress on health disease prevention and promotion can assist in moving us toward becoming a healthier nation.

Most previous research has focused on patient skills and abilities and how to help enhance those skills. As the field of health literacy continues to evolve, there is a growing consensus that health literacy is dependent upon both the skills and abilities of the individuals receiving the health care as well as the professionals providing the care.

However, many professionals and organizations continue to struggle with the concept of health literacy, the implications of low health literacy, as well as the strategies needed to enhance health literacy. The IOM's Roundtable on Health Literacy felt it necessary to commission a paper that would explore what attributes would be necessary for a health care organization to be health literate. A health literate organization is one "that makes it easier for people to navigate, understand, and use information and services to take care of their health" (Brach et al., 2012, p. 2). The paper presented 18 attributes that health care organizations can use as a guide to become health literate and responsive to the needs of the populations they serve.

After obtaining feedback on the abovementioned paper, the workgroup integrated and decreased the number of attributes to 10 and published a discussion paper that, if implemented, will assist organizations to make it easier for individuals to navigate, understand, and use the information and services provided. The 10 attributes should be used as a general guide to embrace the vision of a health literate organization and implement strategies that complement both the resources available and the organizational culture to achieve safe, patient-centered care. The discussion paper was developed so that it could be broadly applied to providers and teams that deliver health care as well as larger health care organizations, payors, and health plans. The attributes should be implemented in ways that align with the needs of each individual organization. As illustrated in Table 5.1, examples are offered as beginning suggestions of how to meet each attribute.

Table 5.1 Attributes of a Health Literate Organization

A Health Literate Organization:	Examples
1. Has leadership that makes health literacy integral to its mission, structure, and operations	• Develops and implements policies and standards • Sets goals for health literacy improvement, establishes accountability, and provides incentives • Allocates fiscal and human resources • Redesigns systems and physical space
2. Integrates health literacy into planning, evaluation measures, patient safety, and quality improvement	• Conducts health literacy organizational assessments • Assesses the impact of policies and programs on individuals with limited health literacy • Factors health literacy into all patient safety plans
3. Prepares the workforce to be health literate and monitors progress	• Hires diverse staff with expertise in health literacy • Sets goals for training of staff at all levels

(continued)

Table 5.1 Attributes of a Health Literate Organization (*continued*)

A Health Literate Organization:	Examples
4. Includes populations served in the design, implementation, and evaluation of health information and services	• Includes individuals who are adult learners or have limited health literacy • Obtains feedback on health information and services from individuals who use them
5. Meets the needs of populations with a range of health literacy skills while avoiding stigmatization	• Adopts health literacy universal precautions, such as offering everyone help with health literacy tasks • Allocates resources proportionate to the concentration of individuals with limited health literacy
6. Uses health literacy strategies in interpersonal communications and confirms understanding at all points of contact	• Confirms understanding (e.g., using the Teach-Back, Show-Me, or Chunk-and-Check methods) • Secures language assistance for speakers of languages other than English • Limits to two to three messages at a time
7. Provides easy access to health information and services and navigation assistance	• Makes electronic patient portals user centered and provides training on how to use them • Facilitates scheduling appointments with other services • Uses easily understood symbols in way finding signage
8. Designs and distributes print, audiovisual, and social media content that is easy to understand and act on	• Involves diverse audiences, including those with limited health literacy, in development and rigorous user testing • Uses a quality translation process to produce materials in languages other than English
9. Addresses health literacy in high-risk situations, including care transitions and communications about medicines	• Prioritizes high-risk situations (e.g., informed consent for surgery and other invasive procedures) • Emphasizes high-risk topics (e.g., conditions that require extensive self-management)
10. Communicates clearly what health plans cover and what individuals will have to pay for services	• Provides easy-to-understand descriptions of health insurance policies • Communicates the out-of-pocket costs for health care services before they are delivered

It is a critical time in health care, a time to shift our perspective from the health literacy knowledge and skills of consumers to the health literacy knowledge and skills of professionals and organizations. Nurses have an opportunity to play a vital role in health literacy awareness, education, and research. Over the past 15 years, there has been a tremendous effort to enhance health literacy through a variety of vehicles, as evidenced by the reports, discussion papers, workshops, and initiatives in Table 5.2. Tremendous opportunities exist for nurses to enhance the patient's experience of care, especially for low health-literate patient populations. The nursing profession is ideally positioned to make a difference and truly impact upon patient-centered care, patient safety, and ultimately, patient outcomes.

Table 5.2 Health Literacy Papers, Reports, and Workshops

Healthy People 2010	2000	Identified health literacy as a public health concern; objectives focused on health literacy
National Assessment of Adult Literacy (NAAL), Department of Education	2003	Established a foundational baseline for future measurement of health literacy
Health Literacy: A Prescription to End Confusion	2004	Definition and conceptual frameworks for health literacy; recommendation to enhance health literacy education in health professionals' curricula and also as continuing education
Surgeon General's Workshop on Improving Health Literacy	2006	Initiated health literacy conversation for strategic planning and coordination with public and private organizations
Institute of Medicine Roundtable on Health Literacy	2006	Brought together leaders from academia, industry, government, foundations, and associations, and representatives of patient and consumer interests who work to improve health literacy
The Joint Commission Report: *"What Did the Doctor Say?": Improving Health Literacy for Patient Safety*	2007	Effective communication is the cornerstone for patient safety; helped establish the connection between low health literacy and patient safety
The Plain Language Writing Act	2010	Promotes clear government communication that the public can understand and use

(continued)

Table 5.2 Health Literacy Papers, Reports, and Workshops (*continued*)

Patient Protection and Affordable Care Act (ACA)	2010	Health literacy is directly and indirectly implied throughout many of the provisions
National Action Plan to Improve Health Literacy; Department of Health and Human Services	2010	Set forth a vision and seven goals to improve health literacy and create a health literate society
Healthy People 2020	2010	Identified improving the health literacy of the population as a topic area
The Joint Commission: Advancing Effective Communication, Cultural Competence and Patient and Family Centered Care: A Roadmap For Hospitals	2010	Assisted hospitals in addressing the non-clinical areas of health care that are essential components of providing quality and safe patient care along the continuum
Health Literacy Universal Precautions Toolkit (Agency for Healthcare Research and Quality)	2010	Toolkit to assist pediatric and adult physician practices to remove literacy-related barriers and enhance patient understanding
How Can Health Care Organizations Become More Health Literate?: Workshop Summary (Institutes of Medicine [IOM])	2012	Defined a health literate organization and presented 18 attributes that health care organizations can use as a guide to become health literate
Attributes of a Health Literate Organization (IOM)	2012	After obtaining feedback from its first paper, decreased the attributes of a health literate organization to 10 and provided rationale and suggested strategies

References

Agency for Healthcare Research and Quality. (2010, April). *Health Literacy Universal Precautions Toolkit.* AHRQ Publication No. 10-0046-EF. Rockville, MD: Author. Retrieved from http://www.ahrq.gov/qual/literacy/index.html

Berkman, N. D., DeWalt, D. A., Pignone, M. P., Sheridan, S. L., Lohr, K. N., Lux, L., . . . Bonito, A. J. (2004). *Literacy and health outcomes. Evidence report/technology assessment No. 87 (prepared by RTI International–University of North Carolina Evidence-based Practice Center under contract no. 290-02-0016).* AHRQ Publication No. 04-E007-2. Rockville, MD: Agency for Healthcare Research and Quality.

Brach, C., Dreyer, B., Schyve, P., Hernandez, L. M., Baur, C., Lemerise, A. J., & Parker, R. (2012). *Attributes of a health literate organization.* Participants in the workgroup on attributes of a health literate organization of the IOM Roundtable on Health Literacy. Washington, DC.

Institute of Medicine. (2006). *Roundtable on health literacy: The first 5 years: 2006–2011.* Washington, DC: The National Academies Press.

Institute of Medicine. (2012). *How can health care organizations become more health literate?: Workshop summary.* Washington, DC: The National Academies Press.

Kutner, M., Greenberg, E., & Baer, J. (2006). *The health literacy of America's adults: Results from the 2003 National Assessment of Adult Literacy.* Washington, DC: U.S. Department of Education, National Center for Education Statistics.

Nielsen-Bohlman L., Panzer, A. M., & Kindig, D. A. (2004). *Health literacy: A prescription to end confusion.* The Committee on Health Literacy, Board of Neuroscience and Behavioral Health, Institute of Medicine. Washington, DC: The National Academies Press.

Office of the Surgeon General (U.S.), Office of Disease Prevention and Health Promotion (U.S.). (2006). *Proceedings of the surgeon general's workshop on improving health literacy.* September 7, 2006, National Institutes of Health, Bethesda, MD. Rockville, MD: Office of the Surgeon General (U.S.). Retrieved from http://www.ncbi.nlm.nih.gov/books/NBK44257

Somers, S. A., & Mahadevan, R. (2010, November). *Health literacy implications of the Affordable Care Act.* Hamilton, NJ: Center for Health Care Strategies, Inc.

The Joint Commission. (2007). *"What did the doctor say?": Improving health literacy for patient safety.* Oakbrook Terrace, IL: Author.

The Joint Commission. (2010). *Advancing effective communication, cultural competence, and patient- and family-centered care: A roadmap for hospitals.* Oakbrook Terrace, IL: Author.

The Plain Language Writing Act. (2010). *Improving communication from the federal government to the public.* Public Law 111-274, 11th Congress. Retrieved from http://www.plainlanguage.gov/plLaw

U.S. Department of Health and Human Services. Office of Disease Prevention and Health Promotion. (2000a). *Healthy People 2010*. Washington, DC. Retrieved November 17, 2013, from http://www.cdc.gov/nchs/healthy_people/hp2010.htm

U.S. Department of Health and Human Services. Office of Disease Prevention and Health Promotion. (2000b). *Healthy People 2020*. Washington, DC. Retrieved November 17, 2013, from http://www.cdc.gov/nchs/healthy_people/hp2020.htm

U.S. Department of Health and Human Services. Office of Disease Prevention and Health Promotion. (2010). *National action plan to improve health literacy*. Washington, DC: Author.

Wolf, D. M., Lehman, L., Quinlin R., Zullo, T., & Hoffman, L. (2008, October–December). Effect of patient-centered care on patient satisfaction and quality of care. *Journal of Nursing Care Quality, 23*(4), 316–321.

Oral Communication

6

Effective Communication and Plain Language

Terri Ann Parnell

A distraught and anxious mother brings her 4-year-old daughter with asthma to the emergency department (ED). The little girl has significant shortness of breath and appears frightened. Mrs. Jones expresses to the staff that she doesn't understand why the inhaler isn't helping her daughter Margaret, despite being in the ED just 2 days ago. "I give Margaret the inhaler just like the nurses told me to," she states. "It just doesn't seem like the medicine is helping her. Margaret uses the inhaler, feels a lot better, and then even goes to her bedroom to rest up and cuddle with her dog, Champ. Before I know it, she is wheezing again. This happens over and over—she is so scared and I am so frustrated. We need a different inhaler!"

The nurse asks Mrs. Jones if this happens after Margaret cuddles with Champ and she replies that it often does. The medicine helps at first and then even after lying down with Champ like a good girl she gets worse again. The nurse asks Mrs. Jones if she recalls the staff telling her to go through her home and remove all asthma triggers or at least keep them away from Margaret? Mrs. Jones states, "Yes—they told me that! I still don't understand why each time I come here you all speak to me about triggers! We don't own any guns and I would never have them around my little Margaret!!!"

While there is no single, generally accepted definition of plain language, often referred to as "living room language," it is a language that when spoken is understandable to the audience, which means that it may need to change depending on who you are speaking with. It is clear, accurate, and to the point. Plain language is beneficial in both oral communication and in written communication. Speaking in plain language is equally as important as writing in plain language. Many of the same principles apply to both but for the purpose of this chapter we will be discussing plain language and oral communication.

Effective Patient Communication

Effective communication is one of the best ways to facilitate a partnership with patients and families, have them be an active participant in their care, and feel that they are valuable members of the health care team. Adherence to prescribed treatment plans and patient satisfaction are enhanced when there is effective patient–provider communication. In a systemic review of the literature on the relationship between patient experience and clinical safety, British researchers reported positive associations between the quality of clinician–patient communications and adherence to medical treatment in 125 of 127 studies analyzed, and also reported that patient adherence was 1.62 times higher where physicians had experienced communication training (Zolnierek & DiMatteo, 2009). Patients who understand more about why they need to follow care instructions are more compliant, which enhances patient outcomes as well as patient satisfaction. Even when there has been effective communication, research has shown that the majority of patients understand and retain only about half of what their provider tells them. In addition, they are also not comfortable asking providers to repeat or clarify the information (Schillinger et al., 2003). Limiting the amount of information, organizing it in a sequential manner, using action-oriented messages, and keeping your instructions clear will assist in enhancing recall. "Chunking and checking" the information will also help in retention. Chunking and checking is when the nurse stops after each item or two and asks the patient to repeat back the information in their own words. This aids in added retention rather than discussing a lengthy amount of information and then asking the patient to repeat back the information at the end. This process also helps to keep the patient engaged and provides a real-time manner of correcting misunderstood information.

There is a tremendous amount of health information and health education that is communicated verbally among patients, their family members, and health care providers. As nurses, we have a professional responsibility to communicate with all patients and families in a way that is understandable. This can be difficult, as nurses often need to communicate very complex information to a diverse group of patients. Effective communication is not just about speaking and listening, but also incorporating cultural and religious beliefs, literacy and educational levels, linguistic ability, as well as taking the context of the communication into consideration. Hence, always taking a patient-centered approach is crucial as it can assist nurses in individualizing the communication to the learner. Patient-centered communication includes all ethical, high quality health care conversations. It is respectful of and responsive to a health care user's needs, beliefs, values, and preferences (American Medical Association [AMA], 2006). Developing a patient-centered approach will enhance the development of a 50/50 partnership and assist in the building of life long patient–provider relationships. In addition, it is crucial from a patient safety and quality care perspective, especially with those patients that are most at risk from impaired communication.

Medical Jargon and Your Nursing Colleagues

Research has demonstrated that medical jargon is widely used during routine medical visits and is linked to patient confusion (Roter, 2011). Unfortunately, it is very likely that a physician will use at least one term that is considered medical jargon in any given patient visit. In addition, it has been demonstrated that patients rate the interaction in a more positive manner when simpler and less complex language is used (Roter, Ellington, Erby, & Dudley, 2006).

It is not uncommon for nurses to also use medical jargon. It is often used in communicating with other nurses on the nursing unit. These are professional communications and therefore considered appropriate; however, one must realize that patients are in close proximity and may misinterpret what you are discussing professionally. For example, a nurse called down the hall to her nursing colleague in her district "Susie, where is the COW?" Now we all are very well aware that "COW" stands for computer–on-wheels, which is the device, used for documentation in the electronic medical record. However, think for a moment of the patient's horror when over hearing you asking where the cow is?

When giving report to the day nurse coming on at the patient's doorway, the nurse going off shift explained that the patient "experienced SOB and the intern was there all night giving Lasix and monitoring him." Of course, the patient was experiencing *shortness of breath* and was being given a diuretic but that patient inquired why he was being called an "SOB." He thought the staff was upset that he "kept the intern there all night" and was referring to him as an SOB.

Another common anecdote is when referring to the "CABG in bed 423." The patient may ask why she is being called a cabbage when we understand that it is an acronym that refers to a coronary artery bypass graft.

Nurses all use medical jargon, but to lay persons it truly sounds like we are speaking a different language. It is important to note that nurses may even need clarification at times. There is so much verbal shorthand that not all nurses are familiar with all terms as they may not be commonly used in all subspecialties. Therefore, for everyone's safety it is crucial to clarify medical jargon with your colleagues as well. Also be sensitive to the fact that medical jargon may not only confuse patients but they may also misinterpret what it is you are saying, which can have a detrimental effect. If it is necessary to use medical jargon, it is best to make an effort to explain the word and meaning to the patient in plain language.

More About Plain Language

Plain language is helpful to everyone—not only persons with limited literacy or linguistic abilities. Plain language incorporates how the information is organized and presented as well as the tone of the message. It is also determines how much information to provide to the patient at one time, which can be a very difficult task. A common phrase in the field of health literacy and plain language is to provide only "need to know" versus "nice to know" information. It can be hard to decide what to include or what to leave out. This means that the nurse should prioritize the "need to know" information and skills the learner must know and master. The background information or extra details that are not "need to know" can be omitted at this interaction and provided at subsequent discussions.

It is also best to begin with what your learner wants to know. This may include more practical day-to-day information or information related to costs. For instance, a nurse was educating a patient about his activity at home for the initial few weeks after cardiac surgery. She sat down, allocated time, and spoke in plain language. She listened and "chunked and checked" the information but felt like the patient wasn't really engaged in the conversation. At the end of the physical activity instructions she spoke about when he could drive and resume sexual activity. She then noticed that the patient physically appeared to relax, his shoulders dropped, his face became less tense, and he seemed much more engaged. It wasn't until he heard about what was important to him that he really began to listen and become an active participant in his discharge instructions. It can be extremely helpful to begin with asking the patient what questions or concerns he or she has before beginning with what is important to the nurse to explain first. This is an example of the adult learning theory by Knowles (1990), which includes that adults are motivated to learn as they experience needs and interests that learning satisfies and that learning is life-centered. In the above example, the return to driving and resuming sexual activity were of immediate concern to the learner and were also very practical information that he could apply in his daily activities.

Use Understandable Words

In health care we have a tendency to use words that are more complex and abstract and that can be difficult for any layperson to understand. In addition, the environment in which we are teaching can be very noisy with lots of activity and interruptions. It is very common to use words such as "preliminary" when referring to test results rather than simply stating that the results are "not final." "Bilateral" is also commonly used instead of saying "both sides." Another term frequently used by nursing and clinicians in health care is the term "benign." The word alone begins to place patients in a panic and it is much clearer to the patient if we instead used the phrase "not cancer" or possibly even stating that the results are "not harmful." And why not simply use the term "germ" rather than speaking about "bacteria" when referring to infections?

When speaking of referring patients to specialists we often throw around terms such as cardiologist, oncologist, or pulmonologist. Explaining that the doctor the patient needs to visit is a heart, cancer, or lung doctor is speaking in plain language that will benefit all patients.

Be Careful With Interchangeable Words

It is also important to be consistent with the words we select when describing procedures, diagnoses, or discharge instructions. For example, when telling a patient they have high blood pressure, it is important to be consistent when reviewing medication instructions. When instructing the patient about dosage instructions for lisinopril, the medication should be referred to as the one for treating high blood pressure rather than stating that it is an antihypertensive.

The same consistency is important when providing instructions for follow-up appointments. It is common for us to state that the patient will need to go to the walk-in clinic in 2 weeks for a follow-up visit. However, when the patient arrives at the address provided, the signage may state "ambulatory entrance" or "ambulatory clinic" rather than "walk-in" clinic. This can be very confusing to many patients.

Consistency in use of terms is an important component of speaking in plain language. If informing a patient that they have experienced a heart attack, the subsequent instructions should refer to the term heart attack rather than stating, "You should eat more chicken and fish now that you have had an MI (myocardial infarction)."

Words That Sound Familiar but Have Different Meanings in Health Care

There are many instances in health care where words are used that sound alike and sometimes may even be spelled the same but have very different meanings than what nonmedical people are familiar with. The example of the mother bringing her daughter into the ED earlier in this chapter illustrates this with the use of the word trigger. An asthma trigger is a substance, condition, or activity that can cause an asthma attack. This definition is very different from many laypersons' reference to a trigger, which most often is the small device that releases the catch and allows a gun to be fired.

Other health care terms in this category are "stool," "dressing," "gait," "appendix," and "balloon" angioplasty. Imagine what a patient may be thinking if told he is going downstairs to get a balloon angioplasty? Or the story shared by a nurse who was teaching a small group class of outpatients about Coumadin. The nurse was explaining to the participants the importance of assessing for bleeding and mentioned to check the color of their urine and stool. After the class, one of the participants came up to him and said he was remodeling his bathroom and asked what color "stool" he should buy.

Use of Positive and Negative

An important consideration when speaking in plain language is to avoid confusion when providing patients with negative instructions or mixing the message that you are sending. Unfortunately, patients often recall the instructions incorrectly especially if it is new to them and if they do not have it written down. For example, when instructing your patient, "Do not take this pill with milk," the patient may actually remember it as "Take this pill with milk." It may be less confusing to the patient to state, "Take this pill only with water or juice." Whenever it is possible, try to communicate to the patient the instructions that should be done (positive) rather than what he or she should avoid doing (negative). Of course, in certain situations, it may be extremely important to emphasize a particular activity to avoid.

Positive and negative outcomes or results are often very different in the health care setting as well. Informing a pregnant mom that her amniocentesis results came back positive may at first seem like good news to her. The same may be true of a young teenager hearing that the HIV results came back positive. A similar and public example of this was back in 2000, when the former Mayor of New York City was diagnosed with prostate cancer. He had a routine screening test and then a prostate biopsy. In an interview some time afterwards, he shared that he was a bit confused at first by the "positive biopsy result." In this situation, a positive result meant cancer was found. He is a well-educated man, but at first was confused and thought positive was a good result.

Even well-educated persons with no medical background may assume that positive is a favorable or good result and negative is unfavorable or bad result, which is not always the case in medicine.

Avoid the Use of Idioms

An idiom is a combination of words that has a figurative meaning and cannot be understood from the meanings of its separate words but that has a meaning all its own (*Merriam-Webster Dictionary*, 2013). The phrases mean something very different from the literal meaning of the actual words. Examples of idioms commonly used are "I want to give you a 'heads up' about the time for your surgery," "break a leg" when wishing someone good luck, or telling a family member that the scheduled surgery for their relative is routine and should be "a piece of cake," meaning uneventful and routine. Another very common English idiom is "you can't judge a book by its cover." When speaking to patients in plain language, it is best not to use idioms as they may have different meanings to persons from other generations, countries, religions, or cultures.

Concepts Can Be Difficult to Grasp

There are certain concepts or words that are commonly used in health care that can be difficult for patients to understand. Your patient may be familiar with the term but not have the contextual knowledge or experience to truly understand the intent or meaning in the health-related situation that is being referenced. General concepts such as prevention, wellness, and overall health status are examples of very broad concepts that may be difficult for patients and their families to understand. In addition, even if understood, the meaning can be quite different from one person to another. Wellness to one person may mean not being sick and to another it may mean getting enough sleep at night and waking up feeling rested. If using general concepts, it is imperative to define exactly what you mean, personalize it to your patient, and have the patient teach-back what was explained to be certain it was understood as intended.

The concepts of benefit and risk are also difficult as they can be vague and hard to pin down. Therefore, when speaking about benefit and risk it is important to be as concrete as possible. The time frame of the proposed risk is an important aspect to discuss. In addition, thought should be given to whether the risk is discussed in the positive or negative presentation. For example, if in a positive way, a nurse may say, "about 80% of patients go home 3 days after the procedure." Stating this same risk in a negative way would be saying, "about 20% of patients stay longer than 3 days after the procedure." Individualizing the teaching to your patient will be of great assistance and help determine the best way to present risk.

Another concept that can be difficult when discussing risk and benefit is whether it is relative risk or absolute risk. Many people do not understand the difference. Relative risk is more of a comparison such as "you will be three times as likely to feel better after this procedure than if you took only medications." Absolute risk is presented to the patient numerically. An example of absolute risk is stating to your patient, "Two out of 10 patients feel better after this procedure."

Words like "probable," "rarely," "commonly," and "unremarkable" are also difficult concepts for patients to fully understand. For example, when using the term probable, most patients assume this means they will be fine. When using the term "rarely" they may mistakenly interpret it as no risk whatsoever. These conceptual terms need to be clarified so that patients can truly understand the intent and can make informed decisions about their care.

Acronyms and Abbreviations

Acronym use is quite common in the health care setting. To confuse the situation even further, sometimes the acronym is pronounced by stating the individual letters like AAA (A-A-A or triple A) or C-H-F, while other acronyms are pronounced like it was a new word such as PET (pet) scan or CABG (cabbage).

Many acronyms are stated as a single word such as in the example above of PET scan or CABG. Another example is HIPAA, the Health Insurance Portability and Accountability Act. We don't refer to this acronym as H-I-P-A-A, but rather pronounce it as a new word "hip-pa." Similar to PET (positron emission tomography) scan, we also refer to a CAT (computed axial tomography) scan as a cat scan, not a C-A-T scan.

Other common examples are when nurses refer to other areas of the hospital. It is quite common language for staff providing report to each other or when transferring a patient, but very unfamiliar to the patient and family. Some common examples are the MICU—said as "mick-you," PICU stated as "pick-you," and SICU spoken like "sick-you." This may as well be a language other than English because that is how it feels to patients. Imagine for a moment not being in health care and a nurse telling you "we are going to move you from this room to the 'sick-you' to be monitored more closely." How scary would that be?

Acronyms can also have different meanings depending on the reference and if a patient is not familiar with the medical field they may misinterpret the meaning of the acronym. This can cause confusion for the patient. For example, AKA means "above the knee amputation" but to the layperson this more commonly means "also known as."

The acronym AAA stands for abdominal aortic aneurysm in the field of medicine. However, outside the medical field the acronym also stands for the Amateur Astronomers Association, the American Automobile Association, the Appraisers Association of America, the American Arbitration Association, and the American Anthropological Association. Depending on your patient's life experience and previous context, the acronym may have a different interpretation. If we do use an acronym we must be certain that we take the time to explain what the acronym means to the patient so there is no misunderstanding or confusion.

If we use too many acronyms we may overwhelm the patient. Try to limit the number of acronyms used and when possible use the ones that the patient will hear most frequently. For example, if a patient is newly diagnosed with congestive heart failure, the nurse may refer to CHF quite often. After defining what CHF is, she could then use this acronym. Throughout the course of the patient's chronic illness, the patient will probably be hearing the acronym CHF at each physician visit or hospital admission. However, although the patient may hear the other acronyms related to CHF, it may not be appropriate to also use I & O (intake and output) and weights QD (every day).

Alphabet Soup . . .

"When you first come out of the OR you will stay in the RR for a few hours until you wake up, and then will be transferred to the SICU. It is normal for you to have an IV, and frequent blood work like CBCs, and ABGs, to monitor your post op status. The nurse will be checking your BP often so don't be concerned. You will also be connected to a heart monitor because of your history of PAT and AF. The day after surgery you may need another CAT scan to check the surgical site. Before you are discharged you will need to ambulate and have a BM. Please let us know if you need MOM to help you go. On the day of discharge the PA or NP will go over your discharge instructions."

Restating the above paragraph in plain language is not an easy task but imagine how the above information might sound to a patient not familiar with medicine or a health care setting. It probably sounds like a bunch of babble. The nurse could rephrase it so that there is more effective communication. There is no definitive right or wrong as to how to communicate effectively in plain language, as it will change for each patient–provider interaction. Read the paragraph below and see if it appears a bit more understandable. Teach-back would be incorporated at different points in the discussion and clarification would be provided along the way. Visuals would also help with learning such as showing an IV and referring to the heart monitor that patient currently has.

"After your surgery, you will be brought to the recovery room to be closely watched for a few hours. As you become more alert and awake from the anesthesia you will then be moved over to the intensive care unit. This is the area where all patients after your type of surgery are brought. You will notice that you will have an intravenous or IV in your arm. This is to give you fluids and any medicine you may need. The nurses will be taking blood from this IV for testing to monitor your condition after surgery. They will also be measuring your blood pressure. This is routine after surgery, so don't worry that something is wrong. You will also be connected to the machine that records your heart rate like you have now. You may notice beeping and hear other sounds, but please don't worry as it is there to help monitor your heart beat."

Sometimes the doctor likes to have another picture of the area that was operated on to check on how it is healing. He may ask that you have a procedure, where you lie on a table, and a machine moves over you and takes very detailed pictures. This will allow him to see the surgical area from the inside. We will get you up to walk as soon as possible. It is important to help you get back to yourself. You will need to go to the bathroom before you are able to go home. If you feel constipated or cannot comfortably move your bowels please let us know so that we can give you medicine. A member of the health care team will visit with you on the day you will go home to explain your medications, diet and other activity."

Numeracy

There is so much information in health care that incorporates the use of numbers. Numeracy skills are needed when initially selecting a health insurance product and calculating the distance the selected provider is located from where you live, the monthly premium, overall annual cost, and anticipated copayments. Once the provider is selected and a visit is planned, there are numeracy skills needed in establishing how long it will take you to travel the distance by your mode of transportation, what your risk is of a certain disease, how to read nutrition labels to help select the appropriate foods for certain illnesses, and how to calculate costs of and dosage directions for medications that may be prescribed. When having a procedure or being a patient in the hospital, it is common to be asked about your pain "on a scale of one to 10." When discharged from a practice setting or hospital, one may be asked to rate certain aspects of care or communication on a numeracy scale as well. This is a very difficult concept for many persons to process, quantify, and understand.

Health numeracy is defined as the degree to which individuals have the capacity to access, process, interpret, communicate, and act on numerical, quantitative, graphical, biostatistical, and probabilistic health information needed to make effective health decisions (Golbeck, Ahlers-Schmidt, Paschal, & Dismuke, 2005). Golbeck et al. classify health literacy numeracy into basic, computational, analytical, and statistical groupings.

Basic skills are needed when identifying numbers and calculating number of pills to take. Computational includes counting but also quantifying and comparison skills such as deciding on the number of calories per serving from a nutritional label. Analytical health numeracy is needed when discussing percentage, proportion, and estimations such as deciding if your glucose is within a normal range and figuring out how much insulin to take when it is not. Or telling a patient that if he or she decreases his or her weight by 10% it will help the patient's blood pressure and cholesterol. Statistical level of health numeracy is very advanced and these skills are used to comprehend general concepts such as risk and randomization in a research setting (Golbeck et al., 2005).

When educating patients about numbers in regard to measurement, it can be extremely helpful to refer to making comparisons to what is familiar to the patient. For instance, if you want your patient to eat 1 cup of vegetables it may be easier to compare it to the size of a baseball, especially if the patient does not own a measuring cup. Or to limit protein to 2 to 3 ounces, or the size of a deck of playing cards. Of course, if your patient is not a sports fan, a reference to a baseball will not be of much help. We need to always remember to individualize the comparisons to each patient. You may need to make relatable comparisons to other objects such as a CD case, computer mouse, a check book, or ping pong ball.

If discussing discharge instructions with a patient, telling the patient that he or she can lift up to 5 pounds is not helpful to everyone. But explaining that the patient can lift up to 5 pounds, like a 5-pound bag of sugar or flour or a 5-pound dumbbell, will be more helpful depending on familiarity with the object of comparison. Using visual tools, either objects, charts, or pictures, can be extremely helpful in enhancing understanding of health numeracy.

Summary

Nurses can use a number of different techniques to enhance the quality and effectiveness of patient–provider communication. They can use plain language to help communicate more effectively. Using plain language also helps in developing a partnership and engaging the patient in his or her care. Limiting the amount of information and providing only "need to know" information, speaking in plain language, and using visuals to complement the conversation are also useful skills to enhance understanding and outcomes and have patients be active partners in their care.

References

American Medical Association. (2006). *Improving communication–improving care: An Ethical Force Program*™ *Consensus Report*. Retrieved November 17, 2013, from http://www.ama-assn.org/ama1/pub/upload/mm/369/ef_imp_comm.pdf

Golbeck, A. L., Ahlers-Schmidt, C. R., Paschal, A. M., & Dismuke, S. E. (2005). A definition and operational framework for health numeracy. *American Journal of Preventive Medicine, 29*(4), 375–376.

Knowles, M. (1990). *The adult learner: A neglected species* (4th ed.). Houston, TX: Gulf Publishing Company.

Merriam-Webster Dictionary. (2013). Retrieved from http://www.merriam-webster.com/dictionary/idiom

Roter, D. (2011). Oral literacy demand of health care communication: Challenges and solutions. *Nursing Outlook, 59*, 79–84.

Roter, D., Ellington, L., Erby, L. H., & Dudley, W. (2006). The genetic counseling video project (GCVP): Models of practice. *American Journal of Medical Genetics, Part C, Seminars in Medical Genetics, 142*, 209–220.

Schillinger, D., Piette, J., Grumbach, K., Wang, F., Wilson, C., Daher, C., . . . Bindman, A. B. (2003). Closing the loop: Physician communication with diabetic patients who have low health literacy. *Archives of Internal Medicine, 163*, 83–90.

Zolnierek, H. K. B., & DiMatteo, M. R. (2009). Physician communication and patient adherence to treatment: A meta-analysis. *Medical Care, 47*, 826–834.

Role of Culture, Language, and Communication Access Services

Terri Ann Parnell

Case Scenario

Maria R., a 41-year-old, married, bilingual woman, cares for her two young children and works part time at the school. She went to the doctor for a routine annual check up because she was afraid she might be let go because the school was undergoing significant budget cuts. If she looses her job, she will not have health insurance so she wanted to go before the end of the year just in case. After all, it had been about 3 years since her last visit to the doctor.

After the visit, the nurse practitioner was reviewing her lab results and going over a treatment plan to help her lose weight and lower her blood pressure.

"I want to get a better idea of what your activity level is and what type of foods you usually eat. Your blood pressure was a bit high and it would be healthier for you if you lost some weight. Since your last visit you have gained almost 20 pounds. Are you interested in hearing about ways you can help lower your blood pressure and get to a healthier weight?"

"Si, bueno—yes," said Maria. "Okay, good—can you tell me what a usual day is like for you—what kind of food do you eat on a typical day?" "Well, in the morning I usually make sorullo de queso, for me and my children. Entonces, for lunch I eat many different thing. Yesterday I eat cheeseburger, y two soda.

129

Entonces for dinner, I eat arroz y frijoles, con one or two soda. I love arroz y frijoles, mi family eat that every day. Y entonces before sleeping yesterday I eat ice cream for snack. Pero I don't eat that every night," said Maria.

The nurse realizes she is not familiar with the types of foods Maria has mentioned and decides to ask more information so that she can develop a plan for Maria that is culturally sensitive. This will enhance Maria's ability to have effective behavioral and lifestyle changes.

The nurse asks Maria to describe what arroz y frijoles is because she has never heard of this. Maria then explains to the nurse that it is just "rice and beans" in English. Now knowing this, the nurse is able to suggest brown rice as a substitute for Maria's usual white rice, which could be one change to help improve her meal. Possibly beginning to mix both white and brown rice for a less dramatic change at first, and then over time making her meals mostly or entirely brown rice and beans. To enhance effective communication further, the nurse should ask Maria if she would like to speak with her using a free qualified medical interpreter. This would provide for safe, culturally and linguistically appropriate communication and would enhance the patient–provider partnership.

Introduction

As the population of the United States becomes more diverse, the priority of effective communication and providing patient- and family-centered care has been widely agreed upon. Nurses are caring for a wide variety of culturally and linguistically diverse patients and the role of culture, language, and communication access is vital to enhanced patient safety and patient outcomes. Effective communication occurs when both participants comprehend the information discussed and there is opportunity for clarification of the intended message. The Joint Commission (Schyve, 2007) has stated that low health literacy, cultural differences, and limited English proficiency (LEP) are the triple threat to effective health communication. Providing safe, high-quality health care requires overcoming these three obstacles when caring for and communicating with patients and families. Culture, language, and communication access services are vital factors in how health care services are delivered and how treatments are prescribed. Culture shapes how we see value and explain our world, and provides the lens through which we find meaning (Nunez, 2000).

Healthy People 2020 identified an organizing framework that reflects five key areas of social determinants of health (SDOH) including economic stability, education, social and community context, health and health care, and neighborhood and built environment (Figure 7.1) (U.S. Department of Health and Human

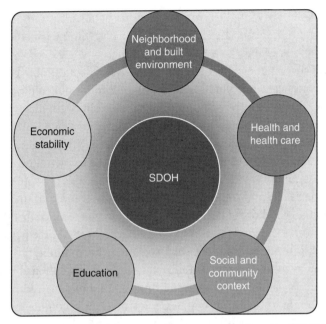

Figure 7.1 Healthy People 2020 social determinants of health (SDOH).

Source: U.S. Department of Health and Human Services. Office of Disease Prevention and
    Health Promotion (2010).

Services [USDHHS], Office of Civil Rights, 2001). Culture, language, and literacy
are included in the SDOH topic area. The topic areas are designed to identify ways
to promote good health for all. Advances are needed in health care as well as other
fields such as education, law, transportation, and community planning to help
ensure that all Americans have equal opportunities to make healthy choices.

Role of Culture

When one thinks of culture and the link to illness and health care, one must
think about the seminal work of Arthur Kleinman from the late 1970s.
According to Kleinman's early work, illness is culturally shaped by how we
perceive, experience, and cope with disease. Our cultural beliefs will determine
how we explain our illness, how we describe our symptoms, who we go to for
care, and what we feel about the care we receive (Kleinman, 1978). Although
there have been many broad and varied definitions of culture, similar themes
have emerged. Culture encompasses beliefs and behaviors that are learned
and shared by members of a group (Galanti, 2007). Culture also includes "the

integrated pattern of thoughts, communications, actions, customs, beliefs, values, and institutions associated, wholly or partially, with racial, ethnic, or linguistic groups, as well as with religious, spiritual, biological, geographical, or sociological characteristics" (USDHHS, Executive Orders, 2013, p. 10). How we view and define health and illness is often viewed through our cultural lens. Each one of us is influenced by our own cultural beliefs, beliefs that may even change over the experiences of our lifetime. It is important to continuously enhance our awareness of the impact of cultural influences upon health and illness.

Leininger's Culture Care Theory of Diversity and Universality (McFarland, 2006) defines culture "as the patterned and valued lifeways of people that influence their decisions and actions." Leininger's theory is directed toward nurses to discover the world of the client and is based on the credence that persons of different cultures can guide nurses to receive the care that these persons need. Nurses must care for their patients with sensitivity and humility as culture and language can affect an individual's understanding and perception of health care.

Cultural awareness is an essential first step in building a foundation for effective communication. Cultural awareness involves becoming aware of our own individual values, beliefs, practices, and perceptions. Take a moment now and reflect on your personal culture. What beliefs do you and your family experience around a particular holiday? How do you celebrate Easter, Diwali, Ramadan, or Passover? What are your specific family traditions? What kind of food do you associate with a particular holiday? What food do you associate as comfort food when you were a child and not feeling well?

I often think about a story shared with me many years ago from a gentleman who was from an Irish family celebrating his first Thanksgiving holiday with a primarily Italian family. All he knew was how he had grown up and celebrated Thanksgiving, which in his particular Irish household meant eating turkey, white potatoes, sweet potatoes, lots of other vegetables, and apple pie and cakes for dessert. When he shared his story of attending his first Thanksgiving celebration with his friend and her Italian family he realized he never thought about how other cultures celebrated the same holiday so differently.

He excitedly arrived for the holiday and soon learned that they served homemade gravy and lasagna with platters of meatballs, sausage, and pork braciole. He said it was so delicious and at the time he assumed they celebrated Thanksgiving with a pasta dinner instead of his traditional turkey dinner, so he indulged in two large servings of the lasagna. To his surprise, the table was cleared and out came several antipasto platters. After the antipasto, the turkey, potatoes, vegetables, bread, and butter arrived. He couldn't believe his eyes and expressed that the food just kept arriving and they sat at the table and ate several courses for hours. After the complete traditional turkey dinner course the fruit platters and fennel were brought out to help with digestion. The evening finally concluded with coffee and espresso, Italian pastries, chocolates, and pies.

Cultural awareness sometimes occurs when we are forced to interact with persons from different cultures or backgrounds. What was considered a "traditional Thanksgiving" celebration for the gentleman in the above story was considered unfamiliar or possibly even inappropriate to a person of a different culture. This story of cultural misunderstanding had no untoward effects except a stomach ache but a lack of cultural awareness can sometimes cause untoward outcomes. Culture is not necessarily conscious and we each must be aware of our own unconscious bias. It is helpful to pause, reflect, and step outside our own comfortable cultural boundaries and become aware of other cultures and learn from and appreciate the differences.

Cultural competence is when patients and providers come together and discuss health concerns without the conversational hinderance of cultural differences (USDHHS, Office of Public Health and Science [OPHS], Office of Minority Health, 2001b). Respecting the health care beliefs and practices of culturally and linguistically diverse patients can help enhance positive health outcomes. Cultural competence begins with reflecting and understanding your own culture and then learning about and understanding other cultures. It is a process of lifelong learning.

In an effort to provide quality nursing care to all patients, nurses must embrace cultural humility. A nurse that practices cultural humility recognizes the limitations of his or her own perceptions and bias and continually strives to be reflective and proactive. Cultural humility should always be present, even when the nurse feels competent in a particular culture. The nurse that practices cultural humility will recognize that his or her own perspective is full of assumptions and will more likely be able to keep an open mind and not feel that his or her way is necessarily the best or only way (Dayer-Berenson, 2011).

Research has shown that cultural differences between patient and provider may not only influence effective communication, but also the decisions the patient makes regarding treatment. When referring to patient–provider communication and culture, it is most common to think about the patient's culture. However, the culture of the provider is also important. When sociocultural differences are not addressed and explored in the interaction, the result is patient dissatisfaction, poor adherence, poor health outcomes, and unfortunately disparities in health care (Flores, 2000). Because of the relationship between culture and health care outcomes, many health care institutions and academic settings across the United States have focused on the development of culturally competent health care professionals. This priority assists in addressing health care disparities in our growing multicultural populations.

One cannot write about the relationship of culture and effective communication, to patient safety, and patient outcomes without discussing the classic book by Anne Fadiman, *The Spirit Catches You and You Fall Down* (1998). This book is both extraordinary and disturbing as it illustrates the contrast between the traditional Hmong culture and the traditional Western medical culture. In this captivating story, both the parents and doctors of Lia Lee, a 3-month-old Hmong girl, wanted the best treatment for her epilepsy (Western diagnosis) or quag dab peg (Hmong diagnosis). Over a period of approximately 4 years, both cultural challenges and linguistic miscommunication exacerbated the collision of these two cultures. Lia's doctors continued prescribing anticonvulsant medication and her parent's preferred their Hmong rituals and animal sacrifices. Lia's parents and doctors all wanted the same positive outcomes for her but were unable to blend the two contrasting cultures. In the research and writing of her book, Fadiman recorded many of her conversations on cassette tapes. She stated in her preface of the book that "she is still learning about both cultures that she has written about and often wonders how the voices on the tapes would sound if she could somehow splice them together, so the voices of the Hmong and the voices of the American doctors could be heard on a single tape, speaking a common language" (Fadiman, 1998).

Enhancing nursing skills regarding the identification of relationships between culture and low health literacy and encouraging the practice of cultural humility will enhance the nurse–patient interaction. If nurses are more aware of the cultural beliefs and preferences of their patient's, they can improve upon the delivery of health care information and services and ultimately enhance patient compliance with prescribed treatments. Roter et al. (1998) summarized results of 153 studies that evaluated the effectiveness of patient education interventions to improve patient compliance and found that combined intervention strategies were more effective than single focus interventions, and that it was crucial that these interventions be adapted with the participant's cultural and linguistic considerations in mind.

"Minority groups currently make up approximately one third of the U.S. population and are projected to become the majority of the population by 2042 and 54% of the total population by 2050" (U.S. Census Bureau, 2008, in the Institute of Medicine, 2011, *The Future of Nursing Leading Change, Advancing Health*, p. 48). Providing staff education in regard to cultural compliance helps develop a mutual understanding and encourage a 50/50 partnership.

However, the approach of cultural competency education is often done with a focus on the differences and specific traditional beliefs or practices of a certain ethnic group (California Health Advocates, 2007). When education is done in this traditional approach, it can promote the tendency to place cultural groups into separate categories; for example, naming beliefs and attitudes of all Asian or all Native American patients and educating about common practices of these groups. However, diversity often exists within cultural groups and there can be much variability even among persons that identify within a similar cultural group. When educating in this categorical fashion, one must be careful to avoid stereotyping of cultural groups as even those with similar cultures may find that they do not share all of the same beliefs, traditions, and practices. Utilizing this global knowledge of a cultural group as a generalization to anticipate your patient's needs can be helpful. If you utilize this general information and first ascertain if it is applicable to your patient, it can assist you in having an informed, open-ended conversation. When learning about a specific cultural group, it is important not to make assumptions or stereotype. Stereotyping can have dangerous negative results. For example, if you believe that all women within a certain ethnic group are extremely expressive and you learn that your patient is from that group, you may underestimate the amount of pain she is experiencing and not offer her pain medication as often as you would another patient that is not in your opinion "typically" as expressive.

Often subgroups or smaller groups of people within a culture have similar characteristics that may not be shared by the larger cultural group. For example, a cultural group I am sure you can relate with is nursing. The broad cultural group of nursing has many subgroups such as medical nurses, surgical nurses, intensive care nurses, or operating room nurses. Ask any nurse and she will tell you that each of these subgroups of nursing certainly have their own cultural norms, beliefs, and practices. We also each belong to numerous other cultural groups related to education, religion, ethnicity, socioeconomic status, geographic location, occupation, gender, age, and many others. Think for a moment of how many cultural groups you actually belong to. We must remember that our patients also belong to numerous cultures and therefore it is crucial that we do not label them within the single culture of their religion, age, ethnicity, disease, or diagnosis. As nurses, we must strive to provide care that is patient-centered and individualized to the patient's cultural beliefs, values, traditions, and practices.

National Standards for Culturally and Linguistically Appropriate Services

The National Standards for Culturally and Linguistically Appropriate Services (CLAS) in Health Care were issued by the USDHHS Office of Minority Health to ensure that all persons receiving health care services receive equitable and effective treatment in a culturally and linguistically appropriate way (USDHHS, OPHS Office of Minority Health, 2001a, p. 3). In April 2013, the USDHHS released enhanced National Standards for Culturally and Linguistically Appropriate Services in Health and Health Care. The enhanced standards are grounded in the broad meaning of culture—one that recognizes that culture is defined in terms of racial, ethnic, and linguistic groups as well as geographical, religious and spiritual, biological, and sociological characteristics (USDHHS, OPHS Office of Minority Health, 2013). The enhanced standards incorporate health and health care organizations and the recipients are inclusive of both individuals and groups rather than patients and consumers from the 2000 standards. The 15 standards incorporate providing effective, equitable, and understandable care and services that are responsive to cultural health beliefs and practices, preferred languages, health literacy, and other communication needs (USDHHS, OPHS Office of Minority Health, 2013). They are not prescriptive and will be implemented differently at different organizations. These enhanced standards are a comprehensive update of the 2000 CLAS Standards and are hoped to be utilized as the roadmap to help organizations improve health outcomes as they continue to care for increasingly diverse communities.

Language and Communication Access

Maria, a 40-year-old Hispanic woman, was having ongoing gynecological issues and had to return to the hospital due to complications. She spoke some English but had difficulty understanding lengthy conversations. Her son was at her bedside when the doctor came in to explain that she would unfortunately now need a hysterectomy as the previously prescribed treatment was unsuccessful. Since he was explaining the upcoming surgery, Dr. Smith wanted to be sure that she understood the risks and benefits so he asked the son to interpret for him instead of depending on her limited understanding of English. After all, he needed to obtain informed consent. Maria unknowingly ended up signing consent for an emergent hysterectomy because her son was embarrassed to interpret to his mother about her "private parts." He was uncomfortable telling Dr. Smith that he didn't want to interpret this sensitive subject to his mother as the doctor was an educated elder and he did not want to appear disrespectful.

Limited English Proficient Persons

Persons with LEP are "unable to communicate effectively in English because their primary language is not English and they do not have fluency in the English language" (USDHHS, Office of Civil Rights, 2001). In the U.S. Census Bureau, persons were asked to report whether they sometimes or always spoke a language other than English at home. It excluded all persons who knew languages other than English but did not speak them at home, who spoke them in a limited fashion at home, or who spoke them in places other than the home. The specific data item was limited to those in the population who were 5 years and older. The data reported that 20.1% of the U.S. population 5 years and older indicated that they were speaking a language other than English sometimes or always at home (U.S. Census Bureau, 2006–2010). When reviewing the data by state (Table 7.1), California reported the most persons (43%) and West Virginia (2.3%) the least persons speaking a language other than English at home.

As the population of the United States that speaks languages other than English continues to grow, providing patient-centered and quality care becomes more complex and challenging. Sixty-three percent of hospitals treat LEP patients daily or weekly, and more than 15 languages are frequently encountered by at least 20% of hospitals (USDHHS, OPHS Office of Minority Health, 2013). Providing health care to meet the needs of the increasingly LEP persons can be challenging, costly, and needs to be coordinated.

Private practices often have limited interpretation services available and financing these services can be a very big challenge to the practitioner. Although the CLAS standards are primarily intended for health care organizations, individual health care practitioners are also encouraged to maintain the same standards and have their practices equally accessible in regard

Table 7.1 Population 5 Years and Over, Percent Speaking Language
Other Than English at Home, 2006–2010

State	Value (%)
Alabama	4.9
Alaska	16.5
Arizona	27.1
Arkansas	6.7
California	43.0
Colorado	16.8
Connecticut	20.6
Delaware	12.2
District of Columbia	14.6
Florida	26.6
Georgia	12.7
Hawaii	25.5
Idaho	10.2
Illinois	21.7
Indiana	7.8
Iowa	6.8
Kansas	10.5
Kentucky	4.6
Louisiana	8.7
Maine	7.1
Maryland	15.9
Massachusetts	21.0
Michigan	8.9
Minnesota	10.3
Mississippi	3.8
Missouri	5.9
Montana	4.6
Nebraska	9.7
Nevada	28.2
New Hampshire	8.0

(*continued*)

Table 7.1 Population 5 Years and Over, Percent Speaking Language Other Than English at Home, 2006–2010 (*continued*)

State	Value (%)
New Jersey	28.7
New Mexico	36.0
New York	29.2
North Carolina	10.4
North Dakota	5.4
Ohio	6.3
Oklahoma	8.8
Oregon	14.3
Pennsylvania	9.9
Rhode Island	20.8
South Carolina	6.6
South Dakota	6.8
Tennessee	6.2
Texas	34.2
Utah	14.2
Vermont	5.4
Virginia	14.1
Washington	17.5
West Virginia	2.3
Wisconsin	8.4
Wyoming	6.7

Source: U.S. Census Bureau (2013).

to culture and language. Standard 4 of the CLAS standards specifically refers to offering and providing free language assistance services, including bilingual staff and interpreter services, to each patient or consumer with LEP at all points of contact in a timely manner and during all hours of operation (USDHHS, OPHS Office of Minority Health, 2001a). In The Joint Commission's publication (2010), *Advancing Effective Communication, Cultural Competence, and Patient and Family Centered Care: A Roadmap for Hospitals*, the need to promote two-way communication is also emphasized.

Language and Communication Interpretation Services

As stated in the National Action Plan to Improve Health Literacy, "everyone has the right to health information that helps them make informed decisions and health services should be delivered in ways that are understandable and beneficial to health, longevity, and quality of life" (USDHHS, Office of Disease Prevention and Health Promotion, 2010). For LEP persons, this means providing all medical information and discussions in an understandable language. The patient–provider partnership begins with identifying a patient's preferred language for discussing health care and raising awareness of any communication needs. Always review the patient's medical record to identify that the patient's communication needs and preferred language for discussing health care are documented.

"Preferred language" is a very important distinction as a patient may be able to communicate in several languages but may prefer one particular language to more easily discuss and understand a medical conversation. At some point in your nursing career you have probably heard a nurse say, "I don't need to use the interpretation services, my patient speaks Spanish but he understands enough English." This can lead to misunderstanding and poor health outcomes. The responsibility is ours to be certain our patients fully understand health information, services, and instructions so they will be more likely to take action and follow treatments that will promote their wellness and health.

The use of medical interpreters is crucial to providing understandable information to LEP patients. Qualified medical interpreters change the spoken word from one language to another, such as from English to Punjabi or from English to American Sign Language for your deaf or hard of hearing patients. Qualified medical interpreters are educated and trained in medical vocabulary as well as ethics, confidentiality, and in maintaining a neutral relationship. It is crucial that hospitals ensure the competency of their language interpreters. The medical interpretation services can be provided in person, through telephonic services, or even video interpretation services.

Oftentimes, untrained bilingual employees or the patients' family members are used to interpret medical information but this should be avoided. This can lead to misunderstanding, errors, and potential legal implications for both the health care professional and the organization. In addition to misinterpreting information, there is also the concern of privacy and confidentiality. It can also be very uncomfortable and even disrespectful to place family members or friends in a situation where they are interpreting medical information that they really should not be involved in.

Interpretation Programs

There are many programs that train and certify interpreters in medical terminology, cultural differences, ethics, and confidentiality. The programs incorporate many hours of education that include medical terminology, oral and written testing, as well as role playing and practicing some typical scenarios they may encounter.

It is not uncommon for the client to become very comfortable with the medical interpreter and sometimes even ask what they think about the situation. The medical interpreter cannot become sympathetic with the client and has to remain neutral and very precise in interpreting the content as it is spoken by the health care professional.

Some helpful tips when using an interpreter include:

- If at all possible, brief the interpreter before beginning. Provide your name and role, and any relevant information to the upcoming conversation such as the purpose of the conversation.

- When communicating with the assistance of an American Sign Language interpreter, the interpreter should be positioned to the side of you and perhaps slightly behind you. This is to facilitate the patient being able to visualize both you and the interpreter at the same time in the same visual field.

- Inform the interpreter that if there is something that is not understood, it should be clarified with you before interpreting to the patient.

- Allow a sufficient amount of time—as the initial discussion is being interpreted into another language it will take at least twice the amount of time and often even longer.

- When speaking, look and speak to the patient and not the interpreter. This is important as there are many nonverbal cues that are important to be aware of during the conversation. It is important to realize that all gestures are not universally understood by all cultures.

- Always speak in the first person. For example, "Mrs. Ortiz, I would like you to stop taking your water pill" rather than saying to the interpreter, "Can you please tell Mrs. Ortiz that she should stop taking her water pill." This will also feel more natural and will help develop a rapport with your patient.
- Speak for a limited time and let the interpreter interpret and then proceed rather than speaking for too long a period of time.

It is important to incorporate the use of "teach-back" just as you would do when communicating with patients in English. Ask open-ended questions rather than questions that require a yes or no response, such as "Mrs. Ortiz, can you tell me how you will explain to your husband how you will take your medications tomorrow? I want to be sure I was clear in my explanation to you."

Effective patient–provider communication is necessary for patient safety. Research shows that patients with communication problems are at an increased risk of experiencing preventable adverse events (Bartlett, Blais, Tamblyn, Clermont, & MacGibbon, 2008). In addition, patients with LEP are more likely to experience adverse events than English-speaking patients (Cohen, Rivara, Marcuse, McPhillips, & Davis, 2005; Divi, Ross, Schmaltz, & Loeb, 2007). All provided language services that meet a patient's communication needs help to promote both quality care and patient safety.

References

Bartlett, G., Blais, R., Tamblyn, R., Clermont, R. J., & MacGibbon, B. (2008). Impact of patient communication problems on the risk of preventable adverse events in acute care settings. *Canadian Medical Association Journal, 178*(12), 1555–1562.

California Health Advocates. (2007). *Are you practicing cultural humility?— The key to success in cultural competence.* Retrieved from http://www .cahealthadvocates.org/news/disparities/2007/are-you.html

Cohen, A. L., Rivara, F., Marcuse, E. K., McPhillips, H., & Davis, R. (2005). Are language barriers associated with serious medical events in hospitalized pediatric patients? *Pediatrics, 116*(3), 575–579.

Dayer-Berenson, L. (2011). *Cultural competencies for nurses: Impact on health and illness.* Sudbury, MA: Jones & Bartlett.

Divi, C., Ross, R. G., Schmaltz, S. P., & Loeb, J. M. (2007). Language proficiency and adverse events in U.S. hospitals: A pilot study. *International Journal for Quality in Health Care, 19*(2), 60–67.

Fadiman, A. (1998). *The spirit catches you and you fall down. A Hmong child, her American doctors, and the collision of two cultures.* New York, NY: Farrar, Straus and Giroux.

Flores, G. (2000). Culture and the patient-physician relationship: Achieving cultural competency in health care. *Journal of Pediatrics, 136,* 14–23.

Galanti, G. A. (2007). *Caring for patients from different cultures* (4th ed.). Philadelphia, PA: University of Pennsylvania Press.

Institute of Medicine. (2011). *The future of nursing: Leading change, advancing health.* Washington, DC: The National Academies Press.

Kleinman, A. (1978). Culture, illness, and care: Clinical lessons from anthropologic and cross-cultural research. *Annals of Internal Medicine, 88,* 251–258.

McFarland, M. (2006). Culture care theory of diversity and universality. In A. M. Tomey & M. R. Alligood (Eds.), *Nursing theorists and their work* (pp. 472–496). St. Louis, MO: Mosby.

Nunez, A. E. (2000). Transforming cultural competence into cross-cultural efficacy in women's health education. *Academic Medicine, 75,* 1071–1080.

Roter, D. L., Hall, J. A., Merisca, R., Nordstrom, B., Cretin, D., & Svarstad, B. (1998). Effectiveness of interventions to improve patient compliance: A meta-analysis. *Medical Care, 36,* 1138–1161.

Schyve, P. (2007). Language differences as a barrier to quality and safety in health care: The Joint Commission perspective. *Journal of General Internal Medicine, 22,* 360–361.

The Joint Commission. (2010). *Advancing effective communication, cultural competence, and patient- and family-centered care: A roadmap for hospitals.* Oakbrook Terrace, IL: Author.

U.S. Census Bureau. (2013). *American community survey, 5-year estimates.* Retrieved from http://factfinder2.census.gov

U.S. Department of Health and Human Services, Executive Orders. (2013). *HHS reaffirms commitment access to all programs and activities by LEP persons pledged.* Retrieved from http://www.hhs.gov/open/execorders/13166/index.html

U.S. Department of Health and Human Services, Office of Civil Rights. (2001). *Limited English proficiency.* Retrieved from http://www.hhs.gov/ocr/civilrights/resources/specialtopics/lep

U.S. Department of Health and Human Services, Office of Disease Prevention and Health Promotion. (2010). *National action plan to improve health literacy.* Washington, DC: Author.

U.S. Department of Health and Human Services, Office of Disease Prevention and Health Promotion. (2010). *Healthy People 2020.* Washington, DC: Author. Retrieved from http://healthypeople.gov/2020/topicsobjectives2020/overview.aspx?topicid=39#one

U.S. Department of Health and Human Services, OPHS Office of Minority Health. (2001a). *National standards for culturally and linguistically appropriate services in health care.* Rockville, MD: IQ Solutions, Inc.

U.S. Department of Health and Human Services, OPHS Office of Minority Health. (2001b). *What is cultural competency?* Retrieved from http://minorityhealth.hhs.gov/templates/browse.aspx?lvl=2&lvlID=11

U.S. Department of Health and Human Services, OPHS Office of Minority Health. (2013). *National standards for culturally and linguistically appropriate services in health and health care: A blueprint for advancing and sustaining CLAS policy and practice.* Rockville, MD: Author.

Nursing Strategies to Enhance Effective Communication

Terri Ann Parnell

"I suspect that the most basic and powerful way to connect to another person is to listen. Just listen . . . . When people are talking, there is no need to do anything but receive them" (Rachel Naomi Remen, MD, Kitchen Table Wisdom).

Every patient–provider interaction is an opportunity for both persons to communicate. Communication is a process by which information is exchanged between individuals through a common system of symbols, signs, or behavior (*Merriam-Webster Dictionary*, 2013). It includes the exchange of information and messages, and is an opportunity for both parties to speak, listen, and understand. Both patients and providers will have different motivations and expertise in their ability to communicate effectively. There are many nursing strategies that can be used to enhance effective communication. The necessary strategies may differ with each interaction depending upon the needs, desires, and skills of the patient. As nurses become more experienced integrating strategies into each communication encounter, they will become more agile adapting their strategies to the needs of each individual patient.

Foster Dignity and Respect

The majority of patients are more comfortable when nurses express a warm, understanding manner and when they let their patients know that their participation is welcomed and even encouraged. Conveying to the patient that they are a valuable member of the health care team is essential in building trust and rapport. Establishing and developing a professional relationship with patients is a crucial part of being professionally accountable.

In the process of caring, nurses receive as well as give (Beeby, 2000). However, it is not always easy to care for and connect to all patients. Patients may be undergoing a tremendous amount of stress, pain, and uncertainty. They may have different beliefs, values, and responses to illness and pain. Being empathetic, caring, and looking at the situation from the patient's perspective can be quite helpful when building a respectful relationship.

Connecting with the humanity of patient's is an essential part of giving and sustaining dignity (Nicholson et al., 2010). Patients maintain their dignity when they feel that their life has value and meaning. When we show respect for our patients we help to preserve and validate their dignity. Research with older adults by Webster and Bryan (2009) demonstrated that older persons value being included in discussions and decisions about their health care. This communication enables them to feel more in control and also helps maintain their independence as well as their dignity. A thoughtful, respectful, and considerate nurse was of great importance.

Everyone is entitled to dignity and respect, and when this is compromised it is a violation to them as a human being. When we do not communicate effectively we are not treating our patients with dignity and respect. Preserving our patient's dignity and respect can enhance effective communication.

Key strategies to enhance dignity and respect include:

- Speaking to our patients in a considerate manner, and utilizing plain language.
- Assessing and making accommodations for the patient's individual communication needs and abilities (language, hearing, speech, cognitive understanding).
- Assessing the patient's baseline knowledge, understanding, and skills.
- Acknowledging the patient's contribution to the proposed treatment plan.

Create a Shame-Free Environment

It is not uncommon for nurses to sometimes forget that the health care setting can be a foreign, uncomfortable, and even frightening environment to those not familiar with the medical field. When we view some aspects of the initial admission experience from the patient's perspective, they unfortunately do not foster a comfortable shame-free environment. Think of the experience from the patient's perspective for a moment—we often ask the patient repetitive questions sometimes in a "rapid-fire" way, we "admit" the patient to a room that is most often shared with a stranger, and then ask them to take the majority of their belongings and personal items and send them home so they won't get lost. The hospital surroundings, sounds, and routine are unfamiliar. Many patients are not able to have family or friends with them and feel alone and vulnerable.

In addition, patients with low health literacy may feel overwhelmed and find it very challenging to answer questions, complete admission paperwork, and sign consent forms. Many patients, including those with adequate health literacy skills, often do not feel comfortable asking questions. They do not want to seem like they are not smart enough or perhaps they feel like they will be bothering the nurse. Educating patients about Ask Me 3® (Figure 8.1), a patient education program from the National Patient Safety Foundation, is an effective approach to encouraging questions and fostering a shame-free environment.

Key strategies to foster a shame-free environment:

- Show respect and a caring, kind manner.
- Introduce yourself and explain your role and purpose.
- Sit down rather than stand whenever possible.
- Orient your patient to his or her room and nursing routines such as visiting hours, time meals are served, pastoral care, rounds, and so forth.
- Ensure a private environment, make eye contact when appropriate, face your patient when speaking.
- Limit distractions and interruptions.
- Ask how the patient would like to be addressed.
- Ask if the patient has any religious or cultural preferences.
- Encourage questions and encourage the patient to let you know if there is something he or she does not understand.
- Offer assistance in completing forms and paperwork.
- Invite the patient to include a family member or friend.
- Encourage patients to ask their health care providers three questions from the Ask Me 3 Program (National Patient Safety Foundation):
  - What is my main problem?
  - What do I need to do?
  - Why is it important for me to do this?

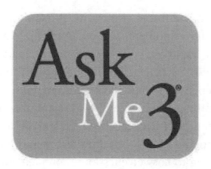

Figure 8.1   Ask Me 3® logo.
Source: Partnership for Clear Health Communication. (n.d.).

Use Plain Language and Speak Slowly

Using plain language purposefully is one of the most important ways clinicians can reduce health disparities related to low health literacy (Sudore & Schillinger, 2009). Nurses should use a "universal precautions approach" and never assume the health literacy level of their patient. Just as nurses wash their hands when caring for all patients, not just the patients that may be at risk for infection, nurses should always speak slowly and use plain, jargon-free, everyday words when discussing medical information with patients. Individualizing the communication and attempting to use words that may be familiar to the patient will enhance the patient's understanding so that he or she can relate on a more cognitive level.

Organizing the information you will be discussing in plain language will also enhance effective communication. It is helpful to first provide an overview of what to expect, such as "First, I will review your activity and then I will go over the written information with you." Ask patients up front what their concerns are and what they would like to know, as these may perceived as most important. Your communication will be patient centered and more effective. Speak with an active voice when addressing patients. For example, "You will take your high blood pressure medicine at breakfast and at dinner." An active voice helps to emphasize the person that will be doing what you are teaching. This is very helpful in personalizing the information and providing clear direction and accountability. Present the information in a logical order and limit the information to as few key points as possible. Although it can be difficult, try to refrain from always being the one speaking. Instead, incorporate silent pauses, even if for just 10 seconds, and really listen to your patient's needs and concerns. This pause allows your patient to think through what you have said, and provides time to collect his or her thoughts. You can encourage your patients to participate more in the conversation by making encouraging comments such as "I didn't know that, I would love to hear more" or "That's really interesting." Asking open-ended questions helps to encourage the conversation rather than a question that can be answered with a simple yes or no. For example, "Can you explain what you think caused your problem?" This conversational style of communicating helps foster a true dialogue rather than a monologue by the nurse with the patient's participation limited to nodding the head throughout the discussion. All patients will benefit from the use of plain language and efforts to engage patients in their health care.

Key strategies when using plain language:

- Speak slowly, clearly, and intentionally.
- Provide an overview of what will be discussed.
- Ask first about patient concerns or questions and what is already known.
- Use everyday words and avoid the use of medical jargon.
- Individualize information by using familiar terms and concepts.
- Allow time to pause and listen; don't be the only one speaking.
- Encourage more dialogue by using encouraging comments.
- Be consistent with word choices—if you use the term "heart attack," don't use "MI" later on in the conversation.
- Use an active voice when communicating.
- Focus your message on behavior or what to do.
- Ask open-ended questions.
- Limit each session to three or fewer key points and repeat when possible.

Assess Learning Styles, Skills, and Preferences

An individual's culture, language, and linguistic ability affect how communication occurs. It impacts the ability to understand and respond in the conversation. This is true for both the provider and consumer of health information.

Recognizing the uniqueness of each person and assessing the cultural beliefs, values, preferences, and attitudes will be extremely helpful in promoting effective communication. Cultural values are the "powerful directive forces that give order and meaning to people's thinking, decisions and actions" (Leininger, 1995). These values and beliefs, of both the provider and the patient, can ultimately affect the process and outcome of learning (Jeffreys, 2010). In addition, words or concepts can differ across different cultural groups. For example, there may not be a word for "psychologist" in your patient's culture or his or her concept of mental illness may be very different than yours. When communicating health information to your patient, it is vital to choose your words carefully and facilitate culturally congruent conversations. Nurses must utilize their resources to effectively meet the challenge of providing health information and educational activities that meet the needs of their diverse patient populations.

When communicating with a person who prefers a language other than English, or who is deaf or has difficulty hearing, it is important to offer free interpretation services and to ask how they prefer to communicate (see Chapter 7, "Role of Culture, Language, and Communication Access Services"). Again, assessing each person's preferred learning style and skills in communicating is essential.

Individuals also have different learning preferences. Although you are communicating orally, it may not be how your patient prefers to learn. It can be helpful to supplement verbal health instructions and information with written material and visuals. Providing visuals or written material is helpful to many patients as it serves as a reinforcement of the conversation. Drawing pictures as you speak can also help illustrate key points and concepts. Using metaphors and stories can assist some patients in understanding or comparing one concept to another, more familiar one. It may even be necessary to read out loud some of the written information used to reinforce the spoken word.

Some people are more skilled at multitasking and managing multiple messages than others. Older adults tend to learn new information at a slower rate than a younger person would due to a decline in reasoning and processing abilities of learning (Beier & Ackerman, 2005). As with all health communication, it is important to take time to assess your patient's learning style and preference and to incorporate and adapt the skills and knowledge necessary to communicate in a respectful, patient-centered manner.

Key strategies to assess learning styles, skills, and preferences:

- Recognize and acknowledge each person's uniqueness.

- Ask how your patient prefers to learn.

- Accommodate and provide language and communication services as needed.

- Choose your words carefully.
- Notice your patient's tone of voice, expressions, and body language.
- Offer paper and pen for note taking.
- Provide written material as a reinforcement of communications.
- Offer to read out loud written information provided.
- Enhance verbal communication with pictures and drawings.
- Incorporate the use of narrative stories and metaphors.

Confirm Understanding

Firstly, I cannot imagine a nurse providing discharge instructions to a patient or teaching about a new treatment and then proceeding to allow the patient to leave knowing that there was no comprehension of what was taught. The biggest misconception is that the nurse or health care provider assumes that what was explained to the patient was understood. After all, the nurse most often asks, "Do you have any questions?" and the patient most often nods "No."

Research has demonstrated that patients recall and understand as little as 50% of what they are told by their doctor (Roter, 2000). Engel et al. (2009) reported that 78% of patients and their families did not thoroughly understand their discharge instructions prior to leaving the hospital. One way to ascertain if your patient has understood what was taught is to ask the patient to repeat back the information in his or her own words. This is a method that is often referred to as the interactive communication loop (Schillinger et al., 2003) or more commonly the teach-back method.

The nurse or clinician would explain the information, then ask the patient to repeat or restate the information in his or her own words. Most often the patient may not recall all that was taught and may benefit from some prompting or clarification. The nurse can re-explain the information, often using different terms or analogies to further enhance comprehension and individualize the content to the patient. The patient would be asked to repeat back again to check for understanding. This process of repeat, clarify, and re-explain would continue until the patient was able to correctly restate the information (see Figure 8.2).

A very important aspect of this process is placing the responsibility of making the information clear and understandable on you. This is not a quiz, and we do not want the patient to feel like he or she is being tested. There are many

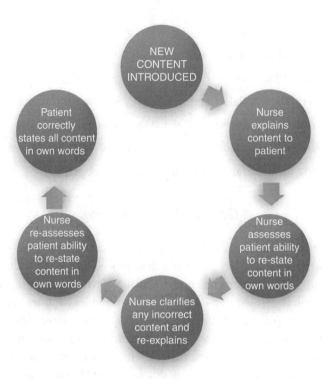

Figure 8.2 Teach-back illustration.

ways to incorporate the process of teach-back in a respectful manner. For example, you might say, "I want to be sure that I was clear in my explanation to you. I
notice your wife is not here with you today; can you tell me how you will explain
this to your wife when you get home later today?" Another suggestion would
be, "We have reviewed so much information this morning. Can you tell me how
you will take your medicine tomorrow? I want to make sure I was clear when I
explained it to you." Or communicate to your patient that "Many patients have
had some trouble understanding this information. Would you mind explaining
to me what foods you will be eating when you get home? I want to be sure I
explained it clearly."

Of course, the way you incorporate teach-back will depend upon each
individual patient context. No matter how you ask your patient to teach-back
the information, it must be done in a comfortable, routine, respectful way. This
will encourage patients to ask questions and further clarify misunderstandings.

Always remember to document the use of teach-back in the patient's medical record along with the patient's response. This is vital so that the other members of the health care team continue teaching and know what areas need to be reviewed. The teach-back method is an effective way to verify a patient's understanding. Studies have shown that using this method improves patient comprehension and also health care outcomes (Kemp, Floyd, McCord-Duncan, & Lang, 2008; Schillinger, Bindman, Wang, Stewart, & Piette, 2004).

Another way to verify that your patient has understood is to inquire about what other questions he or she may have. After using the teach-back method, ask your patient, "What questions do you have?" or perhaps "What would you like to know more about?" Phrasing the question in this way implies that you expect the patient to have some questions and may even help to empower your patient to ask a question or two. When we ask patients "Do you have any questions?" the most common response will be "no" and if we ask "Do you understand?" they often respond "yes."

Key strategies to confirm understanding:

- Incorporate the teach-back method.
- Respectfully ask the patient to repeat back information in his or her own words.
- Take the responsibility for communicating clearly.
- Document the use of teach-back and the patient's response.
- Ask, "What questions do you have?" rather than "Do you have any questions?"

Summary

In practice, nurses can implement a "universal precautions" approach and not assume any person's health literacy skills. They can ask each patient at the point of care, "In what language do you prefer to discuss your health care?" and also ask, "If there are any religious, spiritual or cultural practices that would enhance the experience?" They can always speak in plain, living-room language and use common everyday words that are familiar to the patient. Individualizing the teaching to meet the patient's needs and learning preferences and incorporating and documenting the use of teach-back to ascertain the patient's comprehension are essential. Simply changing the question to "What questions do you have?" rather than asking "Do you have any questions?" will help to encourage and empower patients to speak up and clarify any misunderstandings.

Begin today! If several of these techniques are new to you, take the first step and begin with your last patient of the day or your first patient after lunch. As you practice these techniques and become more skilled and agile, you will find that you will begin to change the way you communicate. You will provide only the "need-to-know" information, in a well-organized, succinct manner. You will begin to "chunk and check" the information provided so that it is provided to the patient in small sections and then confirmed with the use of teach-back after each section. Encourage each other—celebrate the nurses who are health literacy champions. Mentor each other to become more knowledgeable and help each other to develop effective communication skills.

Nurses can truly make a difference in the integration of health literacy as an "always" event. Enhancing effective communication is vital to patient safety, patient satisfaction, and patient outcomes. Nurses are uniquely positioned to enhance effective communication and foster a health literate environment.

References

Beeby, J. P. (2000). Intensive care nurse's experience of caring. *Intensive and Critical Care Nursing, 16*, 151–163.

Beier, M. E., & Ackerman, P. L. (2005). Age, ability, and the role of prior knowledge on the acquisition of new domain knowledge: Promising results in a real-world learning environment. *Psychology and Aging, 20*(2), 341–355.

Engel, K. G., Heisler, M., Smith, D. M., Robinson, C. H., Forman, J. H., & Ubel, P. A. (2009). Patient comprehension of emergency department care and instructions: Are patients aware of when they do not understand? *Annals of Emergency Medicine, 53*, 454–461.

Jeffreys, M. (2010). *Teaching cultural competence in nursing and health care.* New York, NY: Springer Publishing Company

Kemp, E. C., Floyd, M. R., McCord-Duncan, E., & Lang, F. (2008). Patients prefer the method of "tell back collaborative inquiry" to assess understanding of medical information. *Journal of the American Board of Family Medicine, 21*(1), 24–30.

Leininger, M. M. (1995). *Transcultural nursing: Concepts, theories, research, and practice.* Blacklick, OH: McGraw-Hill College Custom Services.

Merriam-Webster Dictionary. (2013). Retrieved from http://www.merriam-webster.com/dictionary/communication

Nicholson, C., Flatley, M., Wilkinson, D. H., Meyer, J., Dale, P., & Wessel, L. (2010). *Everybody matters 2: Promoting dignity in acute care through effective communication.* Nursing Times.net. Retrieved from http://www.nursingtimes. net/nursing-practice/clinical-zones/mental-health/everybody-matters-2-promoting-dignity-in-acute-care-through-effective-communication/5015287. article

Partnership for Clear Health Communication. (n.d.). Ask Me 3 [Web page on the Internet]. North Adams, MA: National Patient Safety Foundation. Retrieved September 11, 2013, from http://www.npsf.org/for-healthcare-professionals/ programs/ask-me-3

Roter, D. L. (2000). The outpatient medical encounter and elderly patients. *Clinics in Geriatric Medicine, 16*, 95–107.

Schillinger, D., Bindman, A., Wang, F., Stewart, A., & Piette, J. (2004). Functional health literacy and the quality of physician-patient communication among diabetes patients. *Patient Education Counseling, 52*(3), 315–323.

Schillinger, D., Piette, J., Grumbach, K., Wang, F., Wilson, C., & Daher, C. . . . Bindman, A. B. (2003). Closing the loop: Physician communication with diabetic patients who have low health literacy. *Archives of Internal Medicine, 163*, 83–90.

Sudore, R. L., & Schillinger, D. (2009). Interventions to improve care for patients with limited health literacy. *Journal of Clinical Outcomes Management, 16*(1), 20–29.

Webster, C., & Bryan, K. (2009). Older people's views of dignity and how it can be promoted in a hospital environment. *Journal of Clinical Nursing, 18*, 1784–1792.

Written Health Communication

7

9

Content Development

Terri Ann Parnell

Written information is used extensively in the health care arena. Since it is so commonly used, there is often a misconception that is easily understood by the intended audience. In fact, there have been numerous studies that have focused on written communication for patients and the public. The overall findings have reported that health materials are generally written at complex levels that far exceed the ability and reading skills of most average high school graduates (Rudd, 2010). Many patients will therefore be unable to understand the information provided or act upon the prescribed treatment plan. They may also have difficulty preparing properly for upcoming tests, procedures, or surgeries. Well-designed, health literate materials can enhance a patient's ability to manage prescribed treatment plans and chronic illness.

Developing written health material and writing health information for a specific audience require a unique skill set. Using plain language to communicate in an understandable way has been described as both an art and a science (Osborne, 2013). Science is necessary as health information and instructions are based on established guidelines, standards, and best practices. The "art" aspect of writing in plain language is necessary as the information needs to be written in an understandable yet pleasing, useful, and relevant manner for the intended audience (Osborne, 2013, p. 157). It can be quite challenging to take complicated medical information and rewrite it into plain language.

Nurses can play an important role and advocate for improvements in health-related written material. They can help identify, review, and revise current written materials as they are most often written at a very high reading level. In fact, many written health education materials are well above the eighth-grade reading level. Rewriting or developing new materials using plain language will help lessen the health literacy burden on all receivers of health information.

Opportunities for Improvement

There are many exemplary patient education materials available; however, there is also current patient education material being written and used that places a significant burden on the person reading it. This makes the information much more difficult to understand and in fact may even confuse the reader.

The most common reasons for this mismatch between material and learner are:

- There is too much information in the document.
- The readability level far exceeds the learner's ability to understand the information.
- The information contains medical jargon that is not defined in plain language.

Before Beginning to Write

Before you sit down and actually start writing your patient education materials, there are a few things to think through in the planning phase.

Identify the Intended Audience

Take a moment to think about who you will be writing this for. If it is a generally applicable topic, first think about why it is important for the learner to read the document.

This will also help you determine what other clinicians or professionals should be involved in writing it. Who are the subject matter experts? What age group or special populations are you writing for? If it is a very specific topic, such as a written brochure on a specific illness, who are the persons most affected by this illness? If the topic is coronary heart disease, the audience would be very different than that for childhood asthma or teenage obesity.

Identify the Goal or Purpose of the Material

It is very important to outline the specific goals of the intended material. What do you want the learners to know by time they are done reading it? Draft an outline with the two or three items that you want the reader to comprehend. Keep in mind, they are the goals of the learner and can be looked at as items you must include in the material. For example, if the instructions are for asthma, the two goals for the patient or learner may be to know what asthma is and secondly, to know how to use the inhaler properly. These must be included in the patient education material.

It is also helpful to the learner when you state the purpose and goals in the beginning of the material before you present it. It "sets the stage" for the learner so he or she knows what to expect. It is also helpful to state the goal or purpose from the learner's perspective, such as, "This information will explain the three activities you will need to do after your hip surgery." When actually reviewing this information with your patient, you can then take the general purpose and make it even more relevant and meaningful to the patient by stating, "These three activities will help you heal so that you can attend your daughter's wedding." This individualizes the information further so that it becomes patient centered.

When formulating the goals of the material, try your best to think of what the majority of the audience or population you are writing for needs to know. Otherwise, your document will contain too much information and become too lengthy.

Guidelines When Developing Written Patient Education Material

Write as if You Were Speaking and Write to the Reader

It is much easier and more interesting to write the patient education material as if you were actually speaking to the reader. Actually, when writing your first outline it is sometimes helpful to write down what you might actually tell a patient. This can assist you to develop your initial outline. This approach is extremely helpful in creating a friendly and personable tone to the content. It also engages the reader, as it will "speak" to them, as they become the person that has to actually "do" what you are asking.

Addressing the reader as "you" helps the user actually picture himself or herself in the content. The information more clearly "speaks" to the reader and can help with accountability. When referring to the reader as "you," it assists in defining responsibility of the behavior change or instructions and can enhance understanding.

Before beginning it is important to think about your audience and the reader of your material. It can also be helpful to draft your outline around the Ask Me 3 questions we teach patients to use.

- What is the main problem?
- What will they need to do?
- Why will they need to do this?

If this feels a bit too restrictive when drafting your outline, you can expand these items a bit further.

- Who is the person that will be reading and learning from your patient education material?
- What does he or she already know about the topic?
- What is it that he or she really needs to know?
- What are some common questions that are asked about the topic?

It can be difficult to narrow down the information to the above outline. As a nurse with so much knowledge and expertise, you will tend to want to include everything while you have the opportunity. Unfortunately, what often occurs is that the patient receives so much written information he or she becomes overwhelmed and even frustrated, and then may not review any of the materials provided.

Write the Information in a Logical, Sequential, or Chronological Order

When writing in plain language, it is very important to not only present the information in a clear, concise manner but also to organize it in a logical, sequential, or chronological order.

Sequential order is slightly different from chronological order and one may be more applicable than another depending upon your content. Sequential order is defined as following a predictable order or pattern while chronological order is ordered or arranged according to the order of time (*Merriam-Webster Dictionary*, 2013). An example of sequential order are the numbering of pages in a book. The pages are ordered in a sequential fashion, page one comes before page two, page two comes before page three, and so on.

Imagine for a moment that you are a chef and are reading a recipe for the first time. You have no experience making this particular item and want to follow the directions as indicated. You would probably first take out all of the ingredients listed in the recipe. Then you may even measure them all out ahead of time. Once you have all of your ingredients you would add and mix them according to the step-by-step sequential instructions in the recipe. If the steps were not listed in sequential order you may not produce the same consistent results and may not be successful with your meal. Listing the steps in a sequential order makes the recipe much easier to follow and also enhances your chances of success. The ordering is an extremely important aspect of the recipe.

In this example, the worse case scenario is that you end up with something that is not edible. Imagine, though, if you were given discharge instructions for changing a wound dressing. The order of how and what you did would make a vital impact on the healing of the wound.

When information is presented in a logical, sequential order, the reader can understand the content a bit more easily. Acting on information that is presented in a disorganized fashion is much more difficult. This is especially true when the information is new to the reader. If you present your content in a sequential, logical order, it is not only easier to understand, but also easier to transition from one step to the next and easier to recall.

If your content does not require an explanation in a step-by-step manner, it is still important to write in a logical sequence. The most important information should be listed or written about first. The reader may not get beyond the beginning of the document, so it is important to write important content up front. More general information should be included before listing out any specific information.

Writing patient materials in chronological order would be appropriate when describing when to take medication or perform a special activity. For example, you would write to "take your vitamin and water pill at 8:00 a.m., then take your stomach medication at 1:00 p.m., and the medicine to help you sleep at 10:00 p.m." Or when drafting a schedule for your patient for wound care, it is best to list the morning, afternoon, then evening dressing changes as it helps the patient to better relate to the timing of the wound care.

Write in the "Active Voice"

When the subject in the material is asked to do something or act, you are writing in the "active voice." Writing in an active voice also helps with accountability, as the reader becomes the subject and the "doer" of the content. It is more difficult to interpret that someone else was supposed to do what was being requested.

Writing in an active voice, also helps to emphasize the requested action. Here are two examples:

Example 1 Active voice: Take your medicine at bedtime.
Passive voice: Medicine should be taken at bedtime.

Example 2 Active voice: Change your dressing every morning.
Passive voice: Your dressing should be changed every morning.

In the above examples, the active voice example emphasizes the action that needs to be done such as "take your medicine" or "change your dressing." Since the active voice focuses on the doer of an action, it is usually clearer, briefer, and more emphatic than when using the passive voice (Center for Plain Language, 2013). Whenever possible, try to use an active voice in your patient education materials.

Make It Understandable and Easy to Read

When writing patient education or health information it is extremely important to write in "plain language" or "plain English." Plain language is communication that is understandable the first time it is read. Written material is considered to be in plain language when the intended audience can:

- Easily find what they need
- Understand what they find
- Use or act upon what they find to meet their needs (Plain Language, 2013)

It can sometimes be difficult to write in plain language. Searching for just the right word can be challenging at times. In addition, when trying to rewrite content in plain language, you must be certain that the intent and meaning of the original message remain the same. It is crucial to have subject matter experts review the document after it is rewritten to ascertain that the information remains on target and is clinically correct.

Define Medical Terms When Used

Whenever possible, try to limit your word choices to shorter words containing fewer syllables. Sometimes it is necessary to use a medical term, as the patient will be hearing this term over the course of his or her chronic illness. In this case, it is important to define the term in plain language the first time it is used. For example, if a patient is newly diagnosed with heart disease, he or she will need to know the medical term cholesterol as this will be monitored on a regular basis. The term should be explained in the written information in plain language. One possible way is by stating that cholesterol is a waxy, fatty substance in the blood that builds up over time on the inside walls of the arteries similar to the build up of grease in the pipes in your kitchen. You can also include a glossary or list of key terms at the end of the document for easy and quick reference.

Avoid Concept and Category Words

Concept words should also be avoided whenever possible. Concept words describe a general idea or an abstract reference (Doak, Doak, & Root, 1996). "Normal," "variety," "frequently," and "often" are examples of concept words that may be misunderstood. When writing in plain language, it is preferable to provide a specific example, such as "exercise three times a week" rather than "exercise frequently." It is a clearer message to write "include two vegetables with your dinner meal each night" rather than "eat a variety of vegetables at dinner."

Category words are terms that refer to a grouping of things. For example, when developing patient education material about a specific diet to follow postoperatively, it is best to write "eat chicken and turkey three times a week" rather than "eat more poultry." Persons with low health literacy may have difficulty understanding the term poultry as it is a category word. Chicken and turkey are very specific and more easily understood. If you choose to use a category word, it is best to then define what you mean after using the term. If the written instructions state, "Eat carbohydrates two times a day." Then you could list several examples of the category term. In this example, "Eat carbohydrates two times a day. Some common carbohydrates are bread, pasta, noodles, rice, or potatoes." The specific examples will help the reader to understand.

Keep Sentences Short and Vary Sentence Length

Sentences should also be kept short and when possible varied in length. Include both short- and medium-length sentences. Avoid the use of complex compound sentences. Group sentences together by topic or idea as it will be easier to comprehend a single topic at a time. If there is a lengthy list of items, you may also want to use bullet points as it creates reading ease and more white space in the document.

Write in the Positive Rather Than the Negative

When writing patient education materials, especially when you want to change behavior, it is best if you can present the information in a positive tone or manner. This is not always possible, but when it is, it is preferable to always explain what the reader can do rather than what they cannot do. Imagine for a moment if you received a sheet of instructions and at the top of the list were all the things you could not participate in. It can be very discouraging and the reader often decides not to read any further. So whenever possible, list what the reader can do and if necessary, follow this list with what they cannot do.

Eliminate Excess Words

When writing patient education materials, there can be a tendency to add words that are not necessary. This can make the message more difficult to understand. Some examples of excess words or commonly used phrases are:

- At the present time—use "now"
- On a daily basis—use "daily" or "every day"
- At a later time—use "later"
- In the event that—use "if"
- Prior to—use "before"

Avoid Medical Jargon and Be Consistent

The use of jargon is common in many professions. Whether it is nursing, medicine, law, engineering, accounting, or dentistry, each profession has its own jargon that is often unable to be understood from those not in the same field. It is taught early in the educational process and in fact, as young students, it is often deemed impressive to rattle off this code language that only classmates can understand.

Fast forward to becoming a practitioner and communicating or writing treatment plans and instructions for patients or clients. Translating this jargon into everyday words can be challenging and may even take practice. In a study of 249 emergency department patients, 79% didn't know that the term hemorrhage meant bleeding and 78% didn't know that fracture meant broken bone, and 45% of the participants were college educated (Lerner, Jehle, Janicke, & Moscati, 2000).

When writing patient education materials it is important to "translate" this medical jargon in more common, everyday words (Table 9.1).

Table 9.1 Plain Language Suggestions.

Instead of	Use
Abdomen	Stomach
Angina	Chest pain
Oncologist	Cancer doctor
Contagious	Spread
Ambulatory	Walk-in
Chronic	Long lasting
Disease	Illness
Erythematous	Red
Mortality	Death
Paralysis	Cannot move

It is also important to be consistent in the words that you use in the written material. If you introduced the word "dressing" in a pamphlet for wound care instructions, don't change the term later in the document to bandage, kling, or gauze. If you used the term "pink eye," don't switch to conjunctivitis or eye infection later on in your writing. The reader may not understand that the words you are using are synonyms but rather may think it is something totally different. This can be difficult to do because when you are writing you will have a tendency to want to interchange different terms for variety in the material.

To Change Behavior, Focus on the Learner

If the intent of your material is to change behavior or enhance a person's skills, that should be the focus of the content. Try not to spend much time writing about the history of an illness or facts about the illness. For example, if developing patient education material about treatment for atrial fibrillation, it is not necessary to begin with when and how the first cardioversion was performed. Or if writing about cholesterol, it is not necessary to include information about how the liver regulates cholesterol levels in the body and synthesizes and exports the cholesterol and helps removes it from the body by converting it to bile. Patients do not necessarily need to know and learn about the underlying principles, anatomy, or physiology in order to change their behavior.

The focus should be on what the learner needs to do, and should be limited to "need-to-know" information that will aid the learner in the changing of their behavior. It is also helpful to highlight the key points or actions in the beginning of the document. The first and last part of the document are often the content that is most recalled—the initial content tends to be remembered the best.

Common Words With Different Meanings

Even when writing in plain language for the health care setting, nurses must be very aware of the words they choose to use. Sometimes in an effort to try and use a more common, everyday word, the word that is chosen may be quite confusing to the patient as it may have a very different meaning outside of the health care setting, even though it sounds the same when spoken and is spelled the same when written. A common example of this when educating in the pediatric setting is the use of the term "trigger." A story shared many years ago was that of a young child that was newly diagnosed with asthma at a clinician visit with her parents. The clinician was investing quite a bit of time teaching the parents about asthma and showing them how to properly position the inhaler on their child's face to administer the medication. The clinician encouraged them to teach-back and even do a return demonstration with the inhaler. Toward the end of the visit, when reviewing all that was taught with the use of the written material, she reminded them to go though their apartment and check for any triggers to help keep their child well. The patient education material referred to "avoid triggers in the home." The mother looked at her husband and said in a rather annoying tone, "Why does she think we have guns in our apartment!"

In this unfortunate scenario, the clinician was well meaning and actually invested a great deal of time and effort in teaching the parents about asthma and the treatment plan prescribed. She even incorporated several health literacy practices such as teach-back and return demonstration. However, upon hearing the term "trigger" from the clinician and reading it in the discharge instructions, the parents immediately assumed that she was referring to guns. The clinician then went on to explain that "trigger" was a term used with asthma and that it was not a reference to guns but meant "factors that can make your child's asthma worse" or "things that can cause an asthma attack." She then provided a few examples that were relevant to the family and their lifestyle such as considering removing the wall-to-wall carpeting in their child's room and leave the hardwood floors exposed with a small, low-pile area rug. She also mentioned that their cat, Sylvester, as a possible cause of asthma attacks due to the pet dander. They also discussed second-hand smoke exposure from their other extended family members that often visit their apartment.

Another example where nurses must be sure to clarify exactly what is meant is when writing information about positive or negative tests results. When writing the terms "positive" and "negative," it is very important to explain it in relation to the context of the topic being discussed in the material. A positive test result could indicate a poor prognosis in some situations and a negative result could refer to a good result. For example, when writing patient education about cardiac testing, when discussing cardiac enzymes it would be preferable to state, "Positive cardiac enzymes mean you have had a heart attack."

Use Visuals—Illustrations, Photos, and Pictures

All persons can benefit from having illustrations that enhance the content in a document, although having pictures can be especially beneficial to readers with low literacy levels. Using visuals in health education materials can increase attention to, comprehension of, and recall of health information, as well as adherence to health recommendations (Houts, Doak, Doak, & Loscalzo, 2006). Visual content in a document can include photographs, pictures, drawings such as anatomical line diagrams, and other images that help to enhance the written content. The illustrations can assist persons in understanding the information quicker and more accurately, as well as help in retention and recall. It is important to try to find the balance between the words on a page and the visuals so that the material is applicable to all audiences regardless of their preferred learning style (Osborne, 2013, p. 215).

It is also best to use pictures that show a positive example or the correct way to perform an activity. This is especially true for persons with low literacy as they may only glance at the visuals and not read the entire text. If your illustrations are of the wrong way to perform an activity or the food you do not want them to eat, often next to content that states not to do this, the content may be misunderstood. Therefore, all illustrations should be of the correct way to do things or of the behaviors you want the reader to participate in. It will also help if you can add a few words to the illustration to aid in understanding. This caption should be placed at the bottom of the picture, and not written across or wrapped around the illustration.

Avoid placing photos or pictures as "fillers" in the document. There are many health brochures that contain a photo of a group of nurses or the health care team, all with smiling faces and all looking like models. While this may be visually pleasing, it is not of much benefit when trying to enhance understanding of the content. It is best to leave more white space and leave the generic photos out of the document.

When selecting visuals to enhance the written content it is important to be certain that what you choose to use is clear to all persons reading the document. Try your best to be culturally sensitive to the audience that will be reading the document. I recall a time when a brochure for a condition called hyperhidrosis was being written and graphically designed. Hyperhidrosis is excessive sweating, most often occurring on the hands, feet, armpits, and groin areas. It often begins in the "tween" or adolescent years, which, as one can imagine, can have significant social and emotional impact upon this age group. The content was written by a subject matter expert, drafted, and designed and was sent to a graphic artist for photos to enhance understanding. The initial photos that came back to enhance the activity section of the content were that of an elderly couple holding hands walking through a park and a middle-aged women playing tennis. These certainly were not relevant to the specific audience for this brochure and were changed to include photos of adolescents participating in different activities.

If the document is intended for a more general population, then a variety of cultures should be represented in the document. It is also equally important when choosing the pictures that they are current and don't have an outdated look to them. If you use outdated photos, the reader will feel that the content is also outdated.

As previously stated, it is best to try to avoid placing too much information about anatomy and physiology as this is often not "need-to-know" information. However, on occasion, it may be important to place a picture or diagram of a specific body part. For example, if explaining about a lung resection, it may be necessary to draw the lung with the lobes labeled so the learner can have this visual of how much of the lung will be removed. If this is the case, it is important to place the picture of the lungs in context with the rest of the body. I recall a time when a patient was a newly diagnosed renal patient and they received patient education information about their upcoming dialysis. There was a drawing of the kidneys next to the content on the page, without any labels or explanation. The picture was inserted to the right of the text and the patient asked "Why is there a picture of lungs over here?" To the patient, the informal drawing of a right and left kidney looked very much like a pair of lungs. It would have been easier for the patient to understand the kidney drawing if they were in anatomical context in the body and labeled. In addition, it can be very disturbing to certain persons or cultures to visualize parts of the body not in correct anatomical placement.

Line drawings can be especially effective when reviewing written material with the learner. For example, when discussing a coronary bypass operation, a line drawing can be very helpful to convey the amount and number of blockages in the coronary arteries as well as where the bypasses will be located. In some written material, it can be helpful to include the basic line drawings of the labeled anatomy and then the nurse can individualize the line drawing when educating the learner. The learner will have the written content, the labeled line drawing, as well as any notes that were written during the education to use for review.

When used correctly, visuals can help enhance understanding of the content, assist in clarifying information, and also help motivate the learner to perform the correct activity or behavior. All readers will benefit from the addition of visuals, but persons with low health literacy skills are more likely to benefit the most.

It's All About the Evidence

Nurses have a vital role when writing health information and educating patients. Evidence-based practice is defined as a problem-solving approach to practice that involves the use of current best evidence in making decisions about patient care (Melnyk & Fineout-Overholt, 2005). When developing and writing patient education, this involves the use of a systematic search for the most relevant evidence and also considers the nurse's expertise as well as the patient's values and preferences (Bennett, 2007). It is the responsibility of the nurse to be certain that the instructions being provided in the written material not only take into account clinical life experience and expertise, but also the evidence from the field to support the document. All patient care must be based upon evidence to ensure patient safety as well as positive patient outcomes.

It's Not Just About Reading Level . . .

When assessing the suitability of the written material there is much more than the readability formulas and grade level. If you have some experience with writing health education materials you may often hear someone ask, "What's the reading level of this brochure?" Or you may have been asked to take a current document and "Make it into sixth-grade reading level."

The history of the most common readability formulas goes back many years and was primarily used to assist educators in selecting textbooks for their students

(Osborne, 2013). They have more recently been used to determine the readability of written health-related materials. Studies have reported that the average adult reads about five grade levels lower than the last year of school that they completed (Doak et al., 1996, p. 28). There are varied opinions in the field as to whether readability formulas should be used in isolation as there are many other aspects in addition to reading grade level that make up the readability of health information. While assessing the readability of a patient-education document with common grade level assessment formulas is a first step, it should not end there. It should actually be just the beginning of evaluating your written material.

Most of the formulas used for readability take into account several factors including the number of syllables per word, number of words per sentence, and number of sentences per paragraph. However, the formulas do not take the meaning of the words nor the order of the words into the calculation. Readability formulas can be helpful in guiding the general evaluation of written health content. In fact, they can be used as a "gut check" to see where you are at as a beginning point, keeping in mind that they only measure a few readability factors. There are also tremendous variations in the interpretation of reading grade level estimates depending on software processing algorithms and the application of each formula (Wang, Miller, Schmitt, & Wen, 2013). In addition, there is a lack of guidelines for the interpretation of these grade level results. The formulas tend to look at punctuation such as periods, bullets, or question marks to determine sentence length. For example, the sentence "Dr. Jones will be in at 12:00 p.m. to check on you." may be interpreted by the formula as four sentences due to the "periods." In addition, in certain online readability formulas, "Xx. Xxxxx xxxx xx xx xx xx:xx x.x. xx xxxxx xx xxx." could be interpreted as the same four sentences but we all know that this is not a complete sentence. Therefore, steps must be taken to prepare your content before analyzing it with the readability formula. Remove bullets and periods that do not indicate the end of a sentence. Also remove headings, subheadings and any titles that you may have on the document so they are not calculated as a short sentence.

There is also variation about whether to remove medical terms that may have been defined in plain language after first use but that remain several times thereafter in the document. If they remain, the reading level would be higher than if they are removed after the initial use and definition. For example, if the term "cholesterol," a four-syllable word, was used and then defined in plain language, some would argue you should remove the term throughout the remainder of the document before assessing readability by a computer program. Others feel it should remain, as you would be falsely lowering the reading level.

A recent study reported that the Flesch-Kincaid formula was the most commonly used readability formula (Wang et al., 2013). The study also reported great variability among formulas—in fact, up to five reading grade levels on the same content—and found that the Simple Measure of Gobbledygook, also known as SMOG, was the most consistent and well matched for health care materials (Wang et al., 2013).

Although there is tremendous variability with readability formulas they can be helpful after the initial draft of a document is complete and then again when you have your final version ready for lay review. It helps to demonstrate to the writer the progress and improvement that was made in the document. However, it should not be the only objective to determine ease of understanding.

Other aspects to look at include many of the items previously mentioned in this chapter. In fact, a content review form or checklist can be quite instrumental in assisting with an evaluation of your written material. The checklist can include both content and design categories. This can be helpful in providing an objective review and evaluation of the material. Most times, the subject matter experts have put a tremendous amount of time and effort into the development of the document. They are not only experts in the particular subject but are also quite passionate about their work. When reviewing material written by a subject matter expert, it is important to not lose sight of the time, effort, and caring that he or she has put into the document and to be especially kind and constructive in your review and critique of the work. A content review form helps to provide objectivity and explanation when reviewing the material for readability. Some of the topics that you may want to include in your content checklist include the following:

- Does the title explain the document?
- Is the material written in a logical order?
- Is the information written in an active voice?
- Is it written in plain language, without the use of medical jargon?
- Are the illustrations and visuals culturally appropriate?
- Does it contain "need-to-know" information?
- Is the information evidence based?

Another way to assess the suitability of material is by using the SAM instrument. This suitability assessment of materials was originally developed and validated by Len and Ceci Doak and Jane Root. It was originally to be used with written materials but has also been successfully used to assess video and recorded instructions (Doak et al., 1996). Utilizing the SAM instrument takes a bit longer, but the more you use it, the more familiar you become with the areas that are scored and the criteria for scoring. The six areas that are evaluated are content, literacy demand, graphics, layout and typography, learning stimulation and motivation, and, lastly, cultural appropriateness. Scoring for each factor is on a scale of 0 to 2 points, not suitable to superior, with a total of 22 factors being scored. If the written material you are evaluating is very long, you can select several areas to score. Each factor contains specific explanations of what the factor should be evaluating. This assists in maintaining objectivity and consistency in scoring with the instrument. After selecting and scoring the material, total the final score and calculate the percentage out of the total possible score of 44 (100%). Then refer to the three categories of percentage ratings:

- 70% to 100% is considered superior material

- 40% to 69% is considered adequate material

- 0% to 39% is considered material that is not suitable

For example, if your total score adds up to 32, the percent score would be 32/44, which is 81% and would be considered superior material. If your total factor score is 26, the percent score would calculate as 26/44, which is 59%, adequate material. Once you have your percentage score, you can decide if the material is suitable or if revisions need to occur.

The suitability of written material involves much more than the reading grade level. The SAM instrument provides a valid process to assess suitability with factors that are not included in readability formulas. A way to enhance this assessment further would be to incorporate lay review with the intended audience.

Incorporate Lay Review to Test Your Document

One of the most important ways to assess if your document is suitable is to ask the reader or intended audience for feedback and clarification that the material is understood. On many occasions, several health care professionals, including nurses and physicians, have reviewed material, and so much valuable information was gleaned from lay review. Surveys or questionnaires that are given to the reviewer are a beginning, but a more robust approach would be an interview or discussion with the reviewer. In addition, the person performing the interview should have an understanding of the purpose of the material being tested. It is not a test, but more a learning session and there are no correct or incorrect answers. It is best to have a person other than the author of the material perform the interview as sometimes the author of the material is so invested in it that he or she finds it hard to be objective and not take the comments personally. Tell your reviewer that you didn't develop the material but are just the person asked to have it reviewed. Also explain that the purpose of the review is to make any changes suggested to make it clear to the reader.

Ask if the material is attractive and inviting, and if the purpose of the message is clear. Can the lay reviewer state and feel as if he or she could follow the key messages in the material? Are all words clear and understandable? Are the photos and illustrations helpful? What does the picture mean to you? Do you feel you can do that, too? Is there anything on this page that you don't like or that your family wouldn't like?

Ask open-ended questions about comprehension of the material. Also try your best not to persuade the reviewer by how you ask the questions. Avoid questions that can be answered with a simple yes or no. It would be best to ask, "When would your family eat this type of food?" rather than "Is this a good picture of a meal your family would like?" The end-user or person representing your audience is truly the expert. The comments and suggestions provided by lay review are invaluable and should be a vital part of written material development.

Telling the Message With Visuals

Many times a story is easier to remember than a list of facts. This approach to developing written materials when educating about health has been especially effective when the message is geared toward a specific population such as educating teenagers about safe sex. The use of fotonovelas is also a popular format to educate about health in a culturally and linguistically sensitive way. A fotonovela is a small pamphlet or booklet, similar to a comic book format, with pictures or photographs and small amounts of text (Flora, 1982; Figure 9.1).

Fotonovelas are a common style of novel among the Latino community; therefore, some health and governmental organizations have adapted this writing style to communicate about health prevention and illness. The development of the fotonovela often includes community partnerships and enhances social experiences. The visuals that are used in this writing style help illustrate a "real-life" experience with which the reader can more easily identify. An educational intervention in a Spanish-speaking Latino community with fotonovelas about

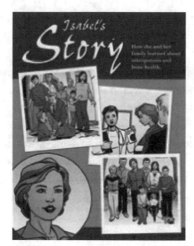

Figure 9.1 Fotonovela about osteoporosis.
Source: http://www.niams.nih.gov/News_and_Events/IRPartners/Spring2007

dementia reported significant learning gains in the 111 participants (Valle, Yamada, & Matiella, 2006). The fotonovela is a successful way of communicating health information as well as other social issues that can affect health indirectly (Kirova, 2008). The use of fotonovelas can enhance understanding, promote empowerment, and even illustrate role modeling for persons with varying levels of health literacy.

Translation of Written Content

Clear written communication is vital to patient safety and for providing quality health care. This is true of materials written in English as well as those translated into other languages. The National Standards for Culturally and Linguistically Appropriate Services (CLAS) in Health Care state that health care organizations must make available easily understood patient-related materials in the languages of commonly encountered groups (Moyer, Guthrie, & Wingert, 2012). Although health care organizations are aware of the existing regulatory requirements, many continue to struggle with the allocation of resources or a formal process for translating patient education in a quality manner.

The translation of English materials into other languages involves much more than simply translating the content word for word into the requested language. After translation into the requested language, there should be a multiple-step process where the intended audience also reviews the document for communicative context in the requested language. In addition, it is important to also review pictures and photos, as they need to be consistent with the culture and customs of the persons who will be reading the information. For example, if you have patient education resource on nutrition being translated into Russian, you would want to change your examples of food preferences into those foods that are commonly eaten by your Russian population.

The Hablamos Juntos ("We Speak Together") initiative, funded by the Robert Wood Johnson Foundation, developed the Translation Quality Assessment Tool for health education materials in an effort to offer health care providers a quality evaluation of a translation product and recommendations on how to possibly enhance communication if there are deficiencies found in the material (Hablamos Juntos, 2009). This assessment tool rates the translated material in four areas, including target language, textual and functional adequacy, nonspecialized content, and specialized content using a four-step rater process. This assessment tool helps to measure how well the translation meets the communicative purpose of the original document while also being sensitive to the needs of the intended language user (Hablamos Juntos, 2009). There is a growing need for quality patent education materials in the multiple languages of the populations they serve.

Tips on Using and Enhancing Existing Materials

What can you do when you have a resource for patient education but you realize that it is not written in the most health literate manner? It is not uncommon to be in this situation, but what should you do? There are a few things you can do to help enhance understanding of written information. You can create visuals to help the reader focus on certain areas of the document and avoid feeling overwhelmed. Some examples of how to create a visual in an existing document would be circling the areas that you want the reader to focus on. To enhance this even further you can then number the circled areas so the reader knows what to look at first, second, and so on.

Other strategies are to underline or highlight key messages in a different color. Perhaps you can highlight the text with a yellow highlighter and number the order you want them to follow. You may also want to use arrows to bring the reader's focus to a particular picture or illustration. To help the reader recall your instructions, you may want to write a short caption under the picture or illustration. Or perhaps the document has photos of what not to eat, which you now know is not the best way to use pictures in a document. You may want to place an "X" through those pictures to remind the reader not to have these food items. The visual clues you use will depend on the document, and the learning preferences of the reader.

Content development checklist:

Did you remember to:

- Write your content for the intended audience?

- Identify the goal or purpose of the document?

- Write using an active voice?

- Place the information in a logical or sequential order?

- Limit the information to "need-to-know" content?

- Limit use of medical jargon or define if used?

- Avoid using concept or categorical words?

- Vary sentence length?

- List the most important information at the beginning of the document?

- Write in the "positive" rather than the "negative" when possible?

- Eliminate all excess words?

- Choose terms and words consistently?

- Define common words that have different meanings in your document?

- Select visuals that enhance your content?

- Assess readability of your content?

- Review your document with the intended audience?

References

Bennett, C. (2007). *Evidence-based practice. Advance for nurses.* Retrieved from http://nursing.advanceweb.com/Article/Evidence-Based-Practice-6.aspx

Center for Plain Language. (2013). Retrieved June 23, 2014, from http://centerforplainlanguage.org/5-steps-to-plain-language

Doak, C. C., Doak, L. G., & Root, J. H. (1996). *Teaching patients with low literacy skills* (2nd ed.). Philadelphia, PA: J.B. Lippincott.

Flora, C. (1982). The fotonovela in America. *Studies in Latin American Popular Culture, 6,* 15–26.

Hablamos Juntos. (2009). *Assessing translation—A manual for requesters.* Retrieved from www.HablamosJuntos.org

Houts, P. S., Doak, C. C., Doak, L. G., & Loscalzo, M. J. (2006). The role of pictures in improving health communication: A review of research on attention, comprehension, recall, and adherence. *Patient Education Counseling, 61*(2), 173–190.

Kirova, A. (2008). Fotonovela as a research tool in image-based participatory research with immigrant children. *International Journal of Qualitative Methods, 7*(2), 35.

Lerner, E. B., Jehle, D. V., Janicke, D. M., & Moscati, R. M. (2000). Medical communication: Do our patients understand? *American Journal of Emergency Medicine, 18*(7), 764–766.

Melnyk, B., & Fineout-Overholt, E. (2005). *Evidence-based practice in nursing and healthcare.* Philadelphia, PA: Lippincott, Williams and Wilkins.

Merriam-Webster Dictionary. (2013). Retrieved from http://www.merriam-webster.com/dictionary

Moyer, D. C., Guthrie, K., & Wingert, B. J. (2012). It's all in the translation. *American Nurse Today, 7*(5), 50–51.

Osborne, H. (2013). *Health literacy from A to Z: Practical ways to communicate your health message* (2nd ed.). Burlington, MA: Jones & Bartlett Learning, LLC.

Plain Language. (2013). Retrieved June 23, 2014, from http://www.plainlanguage.gov/whatisPL

Rudd, R. (2010). Improving Americans' health literacy [Perspective]. *The New England Journal of Medicine, 363*(24), 2283–2285.

Valle, R., Yamada, A. M., & Matiella, A. C. (2006). Fotonovelas: A health literacy tool for educating Latino older adults about dementia. *Clinical Gerontologist, 30*(1), 71–88.

Wang, L. W., Miller, M. J., Schmitt, M. R., & Wen, F. K. (2013). Assessing readability formula differences with written health information materials: Application, results, and recommendations. *Research in Social and Administrative Pharmacy, 9*(5), 503–516.

10

Design Development

Terri Ann Parnell

Every day you can find nurses in facilities and communities, in every specialty, on every shift, educating patients and providing written education materials. Many are also developing their own "home-grown" materials to provide to patients and their families. However, few nurses are well versed in how to properly design the content so that it is health literate. Perhaps the content was written using plain language; however, there are important aspects to design development that can enhance understanding of the information. In fact, you may have written the content using plain language, but when it is drafted, the font is so small that the audience has difficulty reading it, or the contrast between the ink color and the paper makes it difficult to read. Print materials should be written in clear, understandable, plain language, and must also be designed in a way that supports understanding and actually encourages and engages the reader to want to continue to read the entire document. When your document design is done poorly, it can actually detract from the content and even discourage the reader. How you design the layout of the content is just as important as the content itself. This chapter focuses on document design and what you can do to encourage and motivate your readers to want to learn. It is a nursing responsibility to provide information in a way that is understandable so that patients can act upon the information and ultimately enhance health outcomes.

General Concepts

Most written materials have a tremendous amount of time and effort put into them. In fact, when health care professionals take the time to sit down and develop their own materials, I am overwhelmed by their commitment to their patients and to their concern that their patients have the necessary information to care for themselves. It can be quite a difficult conversation, when one has to take this material that was developed as a "labor of love" and explain to the content expert and author that it can be further enhanced so that the patient can truly understand the information. These conversations must be done with a huge amount of respect and sensitivity. If done in this manner, the end result is positive for the content expert and for the patient, as they both will come away with enhanced knowledge.

The most common areas that are often overlooked when content experts first begin writing and designing patient education materials is that they:

- Include too much information
- Write in a passive voice rather than active voice
- Include information about anatomy and physiology
- Use medical jargon and do not define the terms

Format and Layout

User-Friendly Look and Feel

The way a document looks at first glance makes a big difference. If a patient quickly scans a document and it looks and feels overwhelming, it will be tossed aside. Emotionally the patient reacts to the document and tends to avoid trying to decipher the content. On the other hand, if the patient quickly glances at the document and feels he or she can relate and understand the information, it becomes more personal, as if it was written just for that patient. First impressions make a huge difference and how you layout your document can have a tremendous impact on whether your patient decides to invest the time to read through it or toss it aside.

White Space

You may have heard the statement that a document needs to have "enough white space." What this means is that the document should not fill the entire page with words. There needs to be white space, space without words, where the eyes can rest. An adequate amount of white space aids in breaking up the content and also enhances reading ease. I am sure there have been times when you have picked up a paperback book and as you initially flipped through the book you may have noticed that the font appeared very small and the pages were dense with text. I have done this and tended to put the book back down as it can be discouraging at first glance.

However, when there is more white space in the document, it is inviting and enhances the ease of reading the information. How much white space is enough? It will vary from document to document depending on font size and number of pictures, but a general rule of thumb is approximately a 50/50 split between content and white space (Osborne, 2013). Another way to explain this balance is that there should be a 50/50 balance of printed and unprinted sections on each page.

Font Typeface

Selecting the type of font is often a topic of discussion. There are so many to choose from and oftentimes the person who is designing the document prefers to be creative. The author sometimes will use one type font for the title, another for headings, a third for subheadings, and so on. They have the options so they use them! This is another area with general recommendations. Ideally, when writing health information on paper or posters it is recommended to use a serif font. A serif font typeface is one that has the "little squiggly" lines in it or the lines that extend each letter in an upward or downward direction. The main body of text in the document should be in a serif typeface and if you really must be creative, the headings and subheadings can be in one other font typeface. Examples of serif fonts are:

- Times New Roman
- Century
- Palatino
- Garamond

However, if you are designing health information for the web, it is recommended that you use a sans serif font. "Sans" means without, so this is a font that does not have any extra "squiggly lines" or extra strokes at the end of each letter. This helps make the web pages appear more crisp and easier to read, as many computer monitors do not have as good a resolution as paper. If you don't use a sans serif font for web design, your readers may find that the extra strokes or serifs can blur together and make the text harder to read.

Examples of sans serif fonts are:

- Arial
- Century Gothic
- Helvetica
- Verdana

Font Size

Font size is an important aspect. If the document is for a general audience it is recommended to use a minimum 12-point font. Now keep in mind that all font types are not created equal. That is, different font types will vary in size. A 12-point font size is not the same in all font types. See some common examples below.

- This is a 12-point font size in Arial.
- This is a 12-point font size in Verdana.
- This is a 12-point font size in Times New Roman.
- This is a 12-point font size in Chalkboard.
- This is a 12-point font size in Papyrus.

As you can see, each font type is different in size, in height and width as well as closeness of each letter. It is important to know your audience. If designing your content for a specific audience such as a geriatric population or persons with visual impairments, you would want to use a larger font size such as a 14-point font or 16-point font.

Upper and Lower Case Letters

Another common statement in regard to document design is to avoid text in a document that uses all capital letters. It has been said that the evenness of the letters in all capital words makes it difficult for readers of all skill levels. The reading cues that are provided by upper and lower case letters are lost (Doak, Doak, & Root, 1996). Words all have similar shapes, and the height variation in the upper and lower case text assists in the reading of the word.

- AVOID TEXT USING ALL CAPITAL LETTERS.

Notice how the same size in height of the lettering makes it more difficult to read and more difficult to differentiate differences in the words.

- Avoid text using all capital letters.

When writing the same sentence in upper and lower case text, the overall shape of each word varies slightly, which enhances reading. These visual cues are helpful to all readers but especially helpful to persons with low literacy.

- AVOID versus Avoid
- CAPITAL versus capital

If you compare the shape of the word "avoid" or "capital" in the upper and lower case examples to the all capital examples you will notice that the upward and downward extended strokes help change the actual shape of the word. This is extremely helpful to all readers.

Italic or Cursive Lettering

Italicized type is a cursive type of lettering based on calligraphy and often slants slightly upward and to the right (*Merriam-Webster Online Dictionary,* 2013). Italicized letters can get very fancy and ornate and are not familiar to all persons. Designing your document in a font that is more familiar to the majority of readers is more acceptable and also easier for everyone to read. Below are several italicized font types, all in a 12-point font size:

- *Times New Roman Italicized Font*
- *Monotype Corsiva Font*
- *Lucida Calligraphy Font*
- *Mistral Font*

You can see from the selections above that there is a wide range of variability with italic or stylized fonts. Italicized fonts are generally used to bring attention or highlight certain words in a document. If this is the case in a document you are creating, underlining or bolding the word selection will bring the focus to the words while also enhancing principles of plain language.

Paper Choice

After investing so much time writing your content in plain language and testing it with lay reviewers, you don't want to print it on just any old paper. When selecting the paper on which to print your document, it is preferable to use paper with a matte finish to enhance readability for all users. This can sometimes be quite a lengthy conversation if you are collaborating with a marketing team who may feel that glossy paper has a slicker look to it. Paper that has a glossy finish can create a glare that can make reading more difficult. Of course, all matte paper would be the best scenario, but if you must compromise, I would recommend using the glossy paper for the cover of a booklet or brochure and maintain the readability of the information inside the booklet by using a matte finish for the interior pages.

Use of Bullets and Lists

The use of bullets and lists can also help provide visual cues to your readers. If you have a list of items you are instructing your reader about, it is helpful to use bullets to place an extra emphasis or focus on the items. The bulleted list is more visually pleasing as it also provides more white space than if the items were listed in a sentence. The sentence introducing the bulleted list should end with a colon.

For example, if you want your patient to eat more green leafy vegetables it would be visually appealing to bullet the items as in the example below.

- Eat green leafy vegetables such as spinach, kale, collard greens, mustard greens, and lettuce.
- Eat green leafy vegetables such as:
  - Spinach
  - Kale
  - Collard greens
  - Mustard greens
  - Lettuce

Bullet symbols can be solid or transparent circles, squares, arrows, or designs that can even be customized. Again, when selecting the type of bullet to use in a document, one must consider the audience who will be reading it. Select the bullets that appear to reflect the audience, content, and purpose of your document the best. Once selected, it is important to be consistent in use and not have several different types throughout your document.

If the order of your bulleted list is important, it is best to use numbers rather than bullets. This emphasizes the importance of the sequential order of the list for the reader.

Preparing an insulin injection:

1. Wash your hands.
2. Pick up your vial of insulin.
3. If the insulin is cloudy, gently roll the vial between your hands to mix.
4. Do not shake the vial.
5. Wipe the top of the vial with alcohol and let dry.

In this example, the order of the list is extremely important and it benefits from the use of numbers.

Bullets can also help you write your content in a more succinct manner with less redundancy. Rather than repeating words each time, you can begin the list with a statement and then bullet the remaining content. It is also ideal if you can begin the bulleted items with an action verb, underlined in the below example, as it instills a sense of accountability.

- After you are discharged:
  - You should walk two times a day.
  - You should eat three small meals a day.
  - Shower and get dressed each day.
  - Limit the number of daily visitors.

- After you are discharged, every day you should:
  - <u>walk</u> two times
  - <u>eat</u> three small meals
  - <u>shower</u> and get dressed
  - <u>limit</u> your visitors

Try not to have a very lengthy list of bullets. If your bulleted list is becoming too long, you can make it into two columns or perhaps there is a way that you can subdivide the list into subcategories.

- Eat fruits and vegetables such as:
  - Apples
  - Oranges
  - Broccoli
  - Spinach

– Bananas
– Melon
– Carrots
– Turnips
– Tangerines
– Bok choy

Two columns is less overwhelming and visually more appealing.

- Eat fruit and vegetables such as:

– Apples	– Melon
– Carrots	– Oranges
– Turnips	– Broccoli
– Tangerines	– Spinach
– Bok choy	– Bananas

Subdivide the content into two shorter bulleted lists.

- Eat fruit such as:
  – Apples
  – Melon
  – Oranges
  – Bananas
  – Tangerines
- Eat vegetables such as:
  – Carrots
  – Bok choy
  – Turnips
  – Broccoli
  – Spinach

Although bulleted lists assist with placing a focus on important information and are visually pleasing to the reader, one must not overuse them throughout a document. If bullet points are overused or used in an inconsistent manner, it can lessen the impact of their benefits.

Contrast of Paper and Text

Using contrast in your design can be visually appealing to the reader. There are several ways to add contrast in your document. You may want to bold your headings and keep the remaining content in a regular, nonbolded font. Or you may choose to use a different color bullet or bolded bullets to provide visual contrast. While the contrast of black or dark blue ink on white or buff paper provides a pleasing contrast, the opposite would not be true. When designing documents for a general audience it is best to avoid using reverse print. Typically speaking, reverse print would be printing your document with white or light color text on a dark or black background. Although some would state that this also provides contrast, it is difficult to read and would present concerns when printing many copies from a computer or printer.

As with many of the other design elements discussed, using contrast can enhance the readability of your document, but you can overuse a good thing and have an unfavorable outcome. It is not recommended to bold, underline, and use several colors all in one document as it can be a distraction. Select which technique you feel would work best and use that consistently throughout the content.

Justification

Most readers are expecting text that is aligned along the left side of the page with an uneven or ragged right edge. It is more predictable for them and it doesn't distract from the content they are reading (*The Health Literacy Style Manual*, 2005). When words are spaced unevenly it can make reading more difficult. When alignment of the words is not what is expected, it can detract from the content and confuse readers. It is not uncommon to see text aligned differently for design purposes rather than readability. Fully justified, right justified, or centered text can be make it more difficult for the reader of the material. It is best to left justify the content allowing the reader to focus on the content without being distracted by the different design elements. Take a look at the examples below and notice how you feel reading the content. In the fully justified example, take note of the uneven spacing that occurs between words to make the outside edges equally even.

Left justification: Text justified to left, right ragged.

Most readers are expecting text that is aligned along the left side of the page with an uneven or ragged right edge. It is more predictable for them and it doesn't distract from the content they are reading. When words are spaced unevenly it can make reading more difficult. When alignment of the words is not what is expected, it can detract from the content and confuse readers.

Center justification: Text evenly centered, right and left edges jagged.

Most readers are expecting text that is aligned along the left side of the
page with an uneven or ragged right edge. It is more predictable for them
and it doesn't distract from the content they are reading. When words
are spaced unevenly it can make reading more difficult. When alignment
of the words is not what is expected, it can detract from the content and
confuse readers.

Right justification: Text justified to the right, left ragged.

Most readers are expecting text that is aligned along the left side of the page
with an uneven or ragged right edge. It is more predictable for them and it
doesn't distract from the content they are reading. When words are spaced
unevenly it can make reading more difficult. When alignment of the words is
not what is expected, it can detract from the content and confuse readers.

Fully justified: Right and left edges justified, uneven spacing between words.

Most readers are expecting text that is aligned along the left side of the page with an
uneven or ragged right edge. It is more predictable for them and it doesn't distract
from the content they are reading. When words are spaced unevenly it can make
reading more difficult. When alignment of the words is not what is expected, it can
detract from the content and confuse readers.

Select and Place Visuals Carefully

Visuals can have such an important role in enhancing understanding of patient
education materials. When thinking about what types of visuals to use in the
development of your document, it is important to make selections that are
respectful and will not inadvertently be viewed as an insult to a person reading the content. I recall a time when a colleague was developing written patient
education material about stress reduction for patients. The content was developed with a subject matter expert, and then drafted and mocked up. She then
began adding visuals to enhance understanding of the content. One visual that
was added was a cartoon-type picture of an overweight gentleman, with a large
handlebar mustache, smoking a cigar. When the document was sent for lay
review, a comment was shared by the reviewer that it was felt that the cartoon-
type picture she selected to illustrate a person under stress may be insulting
as it may actually look like the reader or perhaps someone the reader knows.

My colleague removed the illustration and replaced it with a visual that was more general and respectful to all. Cartoons should be used with caution and should always be pretested with the intended audience to be certain they are not misinterpreted.

The visual being added should always enhance the content in the document and not simply be placed to look pretty. There have been many occasions when I have seen a document with a picture of a health care team in a huddle, all smiling and looking very attractive. Oftentimes, it is used more as a filler to take up room in the document and does not enhance understanding in any way. In many of these situations, the document would have benefited more if it were left with more white space.

When selecting and placing visuals in your document, the visual should be placed as close as possible to the content it is referring to. When designed in this fashion, the combination of visual and text is helpful to enhance understanding than if one or the other was used alone. Adding a caption with the visual is also helpful in reinforcing the message. In addition, whenever possible, it is ideal to use the visual to illustrate the action or behavior that you would like the reader to perform.

Limit the use of symbols whenever possible as the symbol may not mean the same thing to all audiences. A symbol may not be familiar to all readers and may actually cause more confusion than clarity. If you must use a symbol, it is always best to have it reviewed by the intended audience and have them pretest it to be sure it is clear and understandable.

Table of Contents

In a short or brief patient education resource, a table of contents is not always needed. However, when developing a lengthy patient education document it is helpful to your audience if you provide a table of contents. The use of a general introduction of a few sentences along with a table of contents helps the reader to understand exactly how the information is organized.

Headings and Subheadings

Using headings and subheadings can help to group common items together in one area of the document. Headings can help the reader anticipate the content that is coming and also help the reader organize his or her thoughts

(Doak et al., 1996). It is also helpful when the heading states a complete idea rather than simply a few words.

Header examples:

- Diabetes—The word by itself lacks a complete idea as a header, and is not very inviting or stimulating.
- Diabetes: How to Monitor Your Blood Sugar—This states a complete idea and prepares the reader for the content that he or she will be reading.

Using a question as a subheading can sometimes be successful. The reader can quickly scan through the material to look for the content that is most relevant or to look for the content that is more applicable to them. Using a question as a header can also help to make the material more conversational and interactive as the reader begins to think about the answers (Centers for Disease Control and Prevention, 2009). For example, a heading that states, "When should you call the doctor?" would help a reader quickly find information that would be relevant in an urgent situation. Using headings and subheadings can accurately help the reader learn what will be coming next and also allow the reader to quickly review the material to get a better sense of what is covered in the entire document.

Summary

When developing written materials it is important to write in plain language that is clear and to the point, as this assists in enhancing communication that takes less time to read and comprehend (U.S. Office of Personnel Management, 2013). Writing in plain language assists in enhancing the reader's response to or action from the message. Learning about the intended audience also enhances the ability to clearly direct the format and design in a culturally and linguistically appropriate manner. Asking the intended audience to review and pretest the information helps in providing effective written communication. Good document design enables people to use the text in ways that serve their interest and needs (Schriver, 1997).

Document Design Checklist:

Did you remember to:

- Write in the active voice?
- Leave out anatomy and physiology unless absolutely necessary?

- Avoid use of medical jargon?
- Design with an attractive, friendly look and feel?
- Allow for adequate white space?
- Keep margins at least ½ inch?
- Left justify the content?
- Select a large enough font size with serifs?
- Use upper and lower case lettering and avoid use of all capitals?
- Provide contrast between paper and font color?
- Use bulleted lists when necessary?
- Select visuals carefully and place them near related content?
- Label visuals with captions if needed?
- Include a table of contents if material is lengthy?
- Include headings and subheadings to chunk information?
- Incorporate lay review with your intended audience?

Let's Practice: Before and After Examples

It is difficult to visualize the full impact of the use of plain language and enhancing the understandability of written material when taking small passages and showing before and after examples. There are many factors and variables that enhance the readability and understandability of the written material that are difficult to demonstrate in small excerpts such as the formatting on the page, font size, color, and photos, just to list a few.

Hopefully, you will get a sense and feel for it with a few examples; however, please keep in mind the examples are not complete and are taken out of context.

Before Example 1: Foot Check Program

Kidney failure is often associated with diabetes which can make you less able to find problems with your feet. The dialysis center began a foot check program to help prevent foot problems and to treat them quicker. Therefore, all patients will be asked to remove their shoes and socks so that the dialysis staff can assess their feet for any redness, cracks, or sores. These checks will be done once every quarter, and more often if necessary. Some patients may be asked to see a podiatrist to trim their nails or treat minor problems.

After Example 1

Patients with kidney failure often have diabetes. Diabetes can cause your blood sugar to be higher than normal. This can cause damage to the blood vessels and nerves in your body. When this happens in your feet, it can be hard for you to tell if you have a blister or sore.

- What is the "foot check" program?

  The dialysis unit began a "foot check" program to help prevent problems with your feet. When you come to the dialysis center, you will be asked to remove your shoes and socks. The dialysis staff will check your feet for any redness, cracks, or sores.

- How often is this done?

  Foot checks are done at least once every 3 months.

  If your toenails need to be trimmed or you have a foot sore, you may be asked to see a foot doctor.

Before Example 2

Diabetes is a metabolic disease where you experience hyperglycemia. This can be due to your body not producing enough insulin or your body's cells not responding adequately to the insulin.

After Example 2

Diabetes is a disease or illness where your blood glucose or blood sugar levels are too high. Insulin is a hormone that helps the glucose go into your cells for energy. Glucose comes from the food that you eat. Diabetes can be caused because your body does not make or use insulin well.

References

Centers for Disease Control and Prevention. (2009). *Simply put: A guide for creating easy to understand materials.* Retrieved from http://www.cdc.gov/healthliteracy/pdf/Simply_Put.pdf

Doak, C. C., Doak, L. G., & Root, J. H. (1996). *Teaching patients with low literacy skills* (2nd ed.). Philadelphia, PA: J.B. Lippincott Company.

Merriam-Webster Online Dictionary. (2013). Retrieved from www.merriam-webster.com/dictionary/italic

Osborne, H. (2013). *Health literacy from A to Z: Practical ways to communicate your health message* (2nd ed.). Burlington, MA: Jones & Bartlett Learning, LLC.

Schriver, K. A. (1997). *Dynamics in document design.* New York, NY: John Wiley & Sons.

The Health Literacy Style Manual. (2005). Covering kids and families. Columbia, SC: Southern Institute on Children and Families. Retrieved from http://www.coveringkidsandfamilies.org/resources/docs/stylemanual.pdf

U. S. Office of Personnel Management. (2013). *Plain language.* Retrieved from http://www.opm.gov/information-management/plain-language

IV

Health Literacy and Unique Populations

End-of-Life and Palliative Care

Joanne Turnier

Case Scenario

Joan was a 72-year-old widow who had been living with chronic obstructive pulmonary disease (COPD) for the last 15 years. Joan was placed on oxygen at home and was considered a noncompliant patient. Although she claimed to have stopped smoking, Joan continued to smoke a half of pack of cigarettes every 2 weeks. She believed this was almost as good as quitting because she used to smoke three packs of cigarettes a week.

During the last 2 years Joan experienced frequent COPD exacerbations and was hospitalized a number of times. She refused home care and pulmonary rehabilitation following her discharges. Over the past 3 months, Joan visited the emergency department multiple times and was hospitalized on most occasions. During each hospitalization Joan was intubated and place on mechanical ventilation. With each intubation it became increasingly more difficult to medically wean her off mechanical ventilation. Joan tired quickly and was not able sustain breathing on her own.

Upon Joan's last admission to the medical intensive care unit (MICU), it was evident that she once again needed to be intubated and placed on mechanical ventilation. The medical intensivist told Joan that she would not survive if she was not placed on mechanical ventilation. Given the gravity of the situation, the medical resident approached Joan about her do-not-resuscitate (DNR) status. The resident asked, "In the event your heart stops beating would you like to be resuscitated?" Joan looked upset and stated, "Yes, of course." The resident continued, "Since your condition is getting worse, you will not be able to breathe on your own. We need to place you on mechanical ventilation and this time you may need a tracheostomy. Is there any type of care you would like us to withhold at this point in time? Do you have a living will or a health care proxy?" Joan just stared into space and did not hear a word. She didn't want the resident to know she did not understand anything that he was telling her. She felt so ashamed, and thought "After all this time I should know what the doctors are talking about." The resident continued, "I need to know if you want us to do everything to save your life or would you prefer that we forgo care." Joan stated, "I am having trouble breathing and I want you to do everything to help me to breathe! I get so frightened when I cannot breathe! " Later that morning during rounds, the attending physician and the MICU team discussed Joan's case. Joan was experiencing respiratory distress and her oxygen levels were decreasing. It was inevitable that she would have to be intubated and eventually receive a tracheostomy. This was her last intubation. Joan's lung disease was so severe that she would not be able to live without long-term mechanical ventilation. The social worker was consulted and provided Joan with a list of skilled nursing facilities that accommodated ventilated patients. Joan did not utter a sound as the health care professionals were deciding her fate.

The nurse manager noticed the fear in Joan's eyes and she asked the intensive care unit (ICU) resident to make certain Joan understood her diagnosis and treatment options. The resident asked, "Do you have any questions about what we discussed this morning? You still want us to do everything possible to save your life, right?" Joan nodded yes. The nurse manager wondered if Joan truly understood her diagnosis and treatment options and the consequences of her health care decisions. She did not have a health care proxy or a living will. Joan's brother was listed as her next of kin; however, he lived abroad and would not be arriving until the end of the week. For a number of years Joan was unable to understand, process, and act upon her health information to manage her COPD. The fatal progression of her disease forced her to choose between aggressive life extending treatments or spending the last days of her life in the intensive care unit.

Death in the Intensive Care Unit

Due to the increase in the aging population, more people will die in an acute care setting (Grant et al., 2013). ICUs have become common sites for death in the United States. Approximately 22% of patients die during or after their admission to the ICU (Angus et al., 2004). Barriers to end-of-life care discussions are common in the ICU. Patients and families may have a poor understanding of the patient's diagnosis, prognosis, and treatment options (Levin, Moreno, Silvester, & Kissane, 2010).

The nature of the ICU environment is inconsistent with the philosophy of palliative care (Levin et al., 2010). Historically ICUs are meant to provide highly technical lifesaving modalities. Discussions about withholding or withdrawing life-extending treatments may be perceived as impersonal and inconsistent with the ICU's mission (Levin et al., 2010).

Health care professionals lack the education necessary to address the needs of the dying patient and his or her family (Grant et al., 2013; Levin et al., 2010). The majority of residency programs in the United States do not offer training in palliative care rotations (Billings & Block, 1997; Fisher, Gozansky, Kutner, Chomiak, & Kramer, 2003). Medical students do not feel prepared to enter into end-of-life discussion with their patients (Fraser, Kutner, & Pfeifer, 2001). Even when end-of-life discussions are facilitated through family conferencing, physicians and nurses are often rushed during these communication sessions, leaving little or no time to assess whether the discussion was understood (Levin et al., 2010). Multiple barriers exist in the ICU, making it difficult to address the emotional, prognostic, ethical, and shared decision-making needs of patients and families (Levin et al., 2010). Serious adverse outcomes for bereaved caregivers are evident throughout the literature. Families whose loved ones are cared for in the ICU rather than at home with hospice have five times the risk of experiencing posttraumatic stress disorder and nine times the risk of prolonged grief disorder (Wright et al., 2010)

Physicians and nurses who are constantly exposed to dying patients tend to be more aware of their own mortality, which causes them to have anxiety and emotional discomfort, making it difficult for them to openly discuss end-of-life care (Peters et al., 2013; Savory & Marco, 2009).

Chronic Illness Trends

More than 90 million Americans are living with one chronic illness at a minimum and 70% of Americans will die from chronic illness (Kung, Hoyert, Xu, & Murphy, 2008). Among patients 65 years and older the statistics are even more staggering. Almost 90% of deaths for patients 65 years and older age are directly associated with only nine chronic illnesses which include chronic lung disease, cancer, coronary artery disease, congestive heart failure, renal disease, peripheral vascular disease, diabetes, chronic liver disease, and dementia (The Dartmouth Atlas of Health Care, 2013).

In recent years a significant increase in Medicare spending has occurred as a direct result of the high costs of treating chronic diseases (Thorpe, Ogden, & Galactionova, 2010). Medicare spending (32%) is directly related to physicians' fees and hospital expenses due to hospitalizations from chronic illnesses during the last 2 years of life (The Dartmouth Atlas of Health Care, 2013). It may be possible to reduce spending while improving quality of end-of-life care by ensuring that health care providers adhere to the health care preferences of their patients (Wennberg, Fischer, Skinner, & Bronner, 2007).

Variations in the provision of aggressive care exist across regions throughout the United States. A report from The Dartmouth Atlas Project revealed that the amount of care delivered in a particular region is dependent upon supply and availability of medical resources (Wennberg, Fisher, Goodman, & Skinner, 2008). Due to the uncertainty of how to optimize treatments for patient living with chronic illness, clinicians tend to use resources that are accessible to them (Goodman, Esty, Fisher, & Chang, 2011).

End-of-life care variations are also prevalent across regions. A study conducted by McKinney (2010) examined 235,821 Medicare cancer patients who died between the years 2003 to 2007 and 2010. Patients living in regions where technology is readily available tend to have more visits with physician specialists; some having 10 or more visits during the last 6 months of life. Although fewer patients die in the hospital, those who are hospitalized spend more days in the ICU during the last month of life, nearly 24% from 2003 to 2007 and 29% in 2010. The use of hospice has significantly increased since 2003 in most academic centers throughout the United States. In 2010, 61% of cancer patients were admitted into hospice care compared to 56% in 2003 (Goodman, Morden, Chiang, Fisher, & Wennberg, 2013).

Most patients living with chronic illness have unpredictable prognoses throughout their disease trajectory (Lynn, 2000). Many can tolerate their illness for long periods of time until they are finally overcome by complications that exhaust their already weakened condition (Lynn, 2000). Integrating palliative care is essential when caring for patients with fatal illnesses since there is no way to know which patients are sure to die (Lynn, 2000).

End-of-Life Care

Issues with end-of-life care have been evident for a number of years (Goodman et al., 2011). The Study to Understand Prognosis and Preferences for Outcomes and Risk of Treatment (SUPPORT; 1995) was a seminal study to improve end-of-life decision making and reduce the frequency of a mechanically supported, painful, and prolonged process of dying. The study found that health care providers frequently do not follow their patients' end-of-life preferences. Physicians rarely discuss end-of-life care preferences with their patients and 47% are unaware of their patients' wishes to avoid cardiopulmonary resuscitation (SUPPORT Investigators, 1995). Furthermore, 46% of DNR orders are written within 2 days of death (SUPPORT Investigators, 1995). Despite patients' preferences to die at home rather than in the hospital, most patients still die in the hospital setting (SUPPORT Investigators, 1995).

In 1997, a committee comprised of medical and nursing professionals who cared for chronically ill and terminal patients authored a publication for the Institute of Medicine entitled *Approaching Death: Improving Care at the End of Life* stressing the need for greater access to palliative and hospice care and further encouraged physicians to openly discuss the type of care their patient wanted to receive (Institute of Medicine [IOM], 1997). Four significant findings emerged from the report: (1) suffering at the end of life occurred from health care providers who failed to provide palliative care services; (2) legal, organizational, and economic barriers exist preventing excellent care at the end of life; (3) health care providers lack knowledge to adequately guide and support the practice of evidence-based medicine at the end of life; and (4) end-of-life education and training for physicians and other health care providers are lacking (IOM, 1997). Two additional landmark studies followed the 1997 report: *Improving Palliative Care for Cancer* (2001) and *When Children Die: Improving Palliative and End-of-Life Care for Children and Their Families* (2002). Both reports reiterated the need for evidence-based end-of-life medical care and support for individuals living with terminal illness (IOM, 2001, 2002).

Patient–Provider Relationship: The Importance of Clear Communication

Throughout the past decade, The Joint Commission has stressed the importance of providing safe, quality, patient-centered care across continuums. In 2010, The Joint Commission released a publication entitled *Advancing Effective Communication, Cultural Competence, and Patient and Family-Centered Care: A Roadmap for Hospitals*, in an effort to incorporate concepts addressing communication, cultural competence, and patient- and family-centered care into the fabric of health care organizations (The Joint Commission, 2010). The chapters within the publication highlight six components across the care continuum, including end-of-life care, stressing the importance of addressing the patient's communication needs and monitoring status during end of life (The Joint Commission, 2010). If patient-centered care is to take place, health care professionals must modify their actions to match the skill set of their patient populations (DeWalt, 2007).

For a number of years, the burden of understanding health information has been placed solely on the health care consumer. Health care professionals believed that patients' inability to understand their health information was the only cause of poor health management and outcomes (Koh et al., 2012). Health literacy has evolved into a dynamic, crosscutting issue that not only addresses the patient's knowledge deficits and inability to comprehend health information, but also examines the way health care professionals communicate information to optimize the patient's understanding (Koh et al., 2012).

The complexities of health care delivery systems and the changing demographics create communication barriers especially for vulnerable populations. The elderly, people living with chronic illness, and individuals with diverse cultural backgrounds are at great risk for low health literacy (Kutner, Greenberg, Jin, & Paulsen, 2006; Speros, 2005). Only 12% of English-speaking adults have proficient health literacy skills (Kutner et al., 2006). Low health literacy has serious consequences for individuals trying to manage their chronic illness, which is a key factor in optimizing health outcomes (Doak et al., 2007; Edwards, Wood, Davies, & Edwards, 2012). Patients with limited health literacy have less knowledge and comprehension of their disease and health, reducing their capacity to independently manage their illness and make life-altering health care decisions (Edwards et al., 2012).

Nurses are at the forefront of patient education. It is important for nurses to assess an individual's ability to understand, process, and act upon health care information. This process should be initiated in the early stages of the disease trajectory. Patients living with prolonged chronic illness have an opportunity to build upon their health literacy skills over time. Health literacy encompasses the attainment of knowledge, personal skills, and the confidence necessary to take an active role in self-care and disease management (Nutbeam, 2008). Understanding one's condition is particularly crucial during the last phase of terminal illness. Individuals who have had an opportunity to develop their health literacy skills are better equipped to make life-altering decisions as they approach the final phase of their illness.

The Changing Landscape of Death and Dying

Significant changes in the way Americans die has occurred over the last century. Advances in medical technology and therapeutics have contributed to institutionalization of death (DeSpelder & Strickland, 2010). In the 1900s most people died at home in a familiar environment surrounded by loved ones. In today's world, the dying person is often surrounded by machines and technology, which can indefinitely prolong death (DeSpelder & Strickland, 2010). All too often patients and families want "everything done" to preserve biological functioning without giving any thought to the unintended consequences of their decisions (DeSpelder & Strickland, 2010). The expectation that technology solutions be implemented even when success or cure is improbable has become the norm (DeSpelder & Strickland, 2010). Medical technology has reinforced America's phobia with death and perpetuates the notion that death can be postponed indefinitely (DeSpelder & Strickland, 2010).

The end of life that was once looked upon as a natural progression of a human being's ultimate destiny is now framed by deliberate choices and services provided by the communities of individuals living with terminal illness (Lynn, 2000).

Hospice and Palliative Care

The word hospice was first used during medieval times and referred to a place of lodging and respite for tired, weary travelers (National Hospice and Palliative Care Organization [NHPCO], 2013). In 1948, Dame Cicely Saunders, a British physician, began working with the terminally ill and was the first to apply the name "hospice" to specialized care for the dying (NHPCO, 2013). Saunders's work continued and she subsequently established St. Christopher's Hospice in London, the first modern-day hospice (NHPCO, 2013). In 1963 Saunders introduced the idea of hospice to the United States while visiting Yale University. Her educational sessions to health care professionals and pastoral care providers included visuals of terminally ill cancer patients and their families, illustrating significant positive differences before and after initiating symptom control (NHPCO, 2013). Over the past 40 years, hospice has grown into an enterprise that has served 1.65 million individuals, and 45% of all deaths in the United States were under the care of a hospice program (NHPCO, 2012). Most patients (66.4%) received hospice care at home in private residences, nursing homes, and residential facilities (NHPCO, 2012).

Palliative care extends the principles of hospice care to a broader population that could benefit from receiving this type of care earlier in their disease process. Palliative care ideally would transition into hospice care if the illness progressed (NHPCO, 2013). Palliative care is an approach that improves quality of life for patients and their families facing the problems associated with life-threatening illness through the prevention and relief of suffering by means of early identification and impeccable assessment and treatment of problems, including physical, psychosocial, and spiritual problems (World Health Organization [WHO], 2013).

The need for palliative care continues to grow due to the aging population and an increased percentage of those suffering from fatal chronic diseases. Unfortunately many health care professionals still regard palliative care as terminal care (Morita, Miyashita, Tsuneto, Sato, & Shima, 2009). More often than not, palliative care is restricted to the last weeks or days of a patient's life and utilized only to manage symptoms (Temel et al., 2010). Minimal communication takes place during that time, restricting discussions about goals of care and quality of life. To optimize quality of life, increase survival, and improve emotional well-being, palliative care should be offered as soon it becomes clear that the patient has a chronic, progressive, incurable disease (Temel et al., 2010).

Integration of specialized palliative care teams are successful in addressing physical, emotional, and spiritual distress by providing the patient and family with professional communication that facilitates achievable goals for care and decision making (Meier, 2013). Incorporating palliative care early in the patient's disease trajectory promotes continuity of care and support for the everyday needs of both patients and families across continuums, and reduces hospital cost and the need for ICU hospitalization (Meier, 2013). Patients who received palliative care early in the trajectory of their progressive illness, experienced less depression, have improved quality of life, and survive almost 3 months longer (Temel et al., 2010).

Integrating Health Literacy Into Palliative Care

The Center to Advance Palliative Care recently commissioned a national polling firm to explore the awareness and understanding of palliative care among key audiences and to test language, terminology, definitions, and messaging used in discussing palliative care.

The report provides a detailed look at appropriate messaging and gives insight into the existing consumers' attitudes and perceptions of palliative care (Center to Advance Palliative Care, 2011).

Consumers have no or little knowledge about palliative care—the survey revealed that 70% had no knowledge of palliative care. This confirmed the need to provide consumers with a definition of palliative care that could be understood. Another key finding of the survey was that "language makes a difference" (Center to Advance Palliative Care, 2011, p. 5). It is essential that palliative care be differentiated from hospice or end-of-life care. Confusion among the respondents occurred especially when the terms of "end-of-life care" and "hospice" were included in the definition of palliative care. How health care professionals formulate their discussions made a significant positive difference in the way palliative care was perceived (Center to Advance Palliative Care, 2011).

Once informed, consumers felt positive about palliative care: 95% of the respondents agreed that education regarding palliative care is important for patients and families, and 92% stated that they would be more likely to consider palliative care for a family member if they had a serious illness and shared that it is important that palliative services be made available to patient and families living with serious illnesses (Center to Advance Palliative Care, 2011; Meier, 2013).

Following is a sample of the old language used to describe palliative care in the survey.

Palliative care is the medical specialty that focused on improving the quality of life of people facing serious illness. Emphasis is placed on pain and symptom management, communication and coordinated care. Palliative care is appropriate from the time of diagnosis and can be provided with curative treatment. (Center to Advance Palliative Care, 2011, p. 6)

After being provided with this definition of palliative care, only 36% of the respondents reported that they would access palliative care.

Here is a sample of the new language used to describe palliative care:

Palliative care is specialized medical care for people with serious illnesses. This type of care is focused on providing patients with relief from the symptoms, pain and stress of a serious illness whatever the diagnosis. The goal is to improve quality of life for both the patient and the family. Palliative care is provided by a team of doctors, nurses, and other specialists who work with a patient's doctor to provide an extra layer of support. Palliative care is appropriate at any age and at any state in a serious illness, and can be provided together with curative treatment. (Center to Advance Palliative Care, 2011, p. 6)

Once informed using the new language to describe palliative care, 60% of the respondents said they would be "very likely to consider using palliative care for their loved ones" (Center to Advance Palliative Care, 2011, p. 8).

A Model for Integrating Health Literacy Into End-of-Life Care

Health care providers often overestimate the health literacy skills of their patients, have difficulty recognizing patients with low health literacy, and do not understand the consequences that low health literacy has on health outcomes (Kelly & Haidet, 2006; Kutner et al., 2006). Close to half of the U.S. adult population is unable to understand, act upon, or participate in their health care (Kutner et al., 2006).

Nutbeam (2008) extends the definition of health literacy, viewing it as a "risk factor" moving beyond the notion of intellectual capability, and stresses the importance of integrating communication skills that meet the health literacy needs of individuals. Improving access to health information and teaching individuals how to effectively use it is essential to empowerment (Nutbeam, 2000, 2008). Current definitions of health literacy levels propose measures of achievement in reading and writing; Nutbeam (2000) believes different types of literacy classifications can be integrated into daily activities.

This model of health literacy may address the challenges confronted by patients and families living with chronic progressive illness for a prolonged period of time and may ultimately effect the choices they make in end-of-life care; "such classifications indicate that the different levels of literacy progressively may allow for greater autonomy and personal empowerment" (Nutbeam, 2000, p. 264).

Nutbeam's classifications are broken down into three categories or phases: basic functional literacy, communicative/interactive literacy, and critical literacy. In the basic functional literacy stage, the individual is able to read, write, and function adequately in activities of daily living.

During this phase, it is important to focus on oral and written communication that meets the learning needs of the individual. Nurses are in a position to educate patients about diagnosis, treatment options, and the importance of adherence to the plan of care. Providing clear communication during the initial nurse–patient encounter facilitates a trusting relationship setting, the groundwork for future education. Patients are then afforded the opportunity to develop more advanced intellectual and health literacy skills, which Nutbeam (2000) refers to as the communicative/interactive literacy stage. These skills, coupled with social skills, can be used to increase participation in daily activities. Communicative/interactive literacy also facilitates the individual's ability to extract information and derive meaning from different forms of communication and to apply new information to changing circumstances. The ability to develop communicative/interactive literacy is particularly important during the patient transition from living and functioning with chronic illness to the terminal phase of the chronic illness. Most patients are confronted with life-altering decision making, which may include the decision to forego life extending treatments. This type of decision making requires a deep understanding of the disease trajectory and the consequences of life-altering decision making. With education and support, patient and families are better able to further develop their critical literacy skills, which ultimately advance their intellectual ability. Critical literacy skills can be applied to examine complex information to gain greater control over life events and circumstances (Nutbeam, 2000). Progression through the classification levels is dependent upon the individual's exposure to different information, messaging through the content and method of delivery (Nutbeam, 2000). The method in which the communication is provided depends upon personal and social skills, and the person's ability to complete a task or reach a goal pertaining to the issues discussed (Nutbeam, 2000).

Nurses who care for populations living with chronic terminal illness have an opportunity to help individuals develop and/or enhance their critical literacy skills throughout their prolonged illness, which may facilitate a seamless transition to palliative care. This model provides a framework for nurses to follow as they begin to integrate meaningful communication that empowers patients and families by helping them to overcome structural barriers that interfere with optimizing their health and the decisions they make about end-of-life care (Nutbeam, 2000).

Enhancing Communication in End-of-Life Care

Competence in end-of-life care requires excellent communication skills and the ability to make decisions and to build trusting relationships with patients and families (von Gunten, Ferris, & Emanuel, 2000). Von Gunten and colleagues

(2000) propose a seven-step approach to end-of-life discussions in which the tenets of health literacy can be easily incorporated.

Step 1:   Confirm medical facts and establish an appropriate environment.

Create a shame-free environment. A shame free environment honors the cultural, religious preferences, and decision-making process of the patient and family. Nurses are in a position to learn about their patient's/family's cultural and religious preferences. It is important for nurses to practice cultural humility by respectfully asking questions that assist in gaining a greater understanding of the patient's perception of illness, the cultural and spiritual context, and the role family plays in decision making. Patients and or family members may insist that clergy participate in family conferencing when discussing end-of-life care. It is important for nurses to honor the cultural and spiritual preferences of patients and families.

Step 2:   Establishing what the patient already knows.

Finding out what the patient already knows and eliciting his or her attitude about the illness and or situation provides guidance to nurses in selecting what needs to be discussed and the proper time to discuss it (Doak, Doak, & Root, 2007). It is important to use open-ended questions, illustrations, models, and other visual aids to assess learning needs. Establish the context for asking questions by saying; "I want to discuss your condition with you. Before I begin, I want to be sure I am not taking up your time by providing you with information you already know, so first I will need to ask you a few questions that will help me to know what information I need to give you." The nurse may begin the discussion with "What have the doctors told you about the treatments that are available to you at this stage of your illness?" It is important for patients and families to know why they are being asked questions and how their responses will be used. When patients' know the context, they will better know how to respond (Doak et al., 2007).

Step 3:   Determine how information is to be handled.

Establishing a therapeutic relationship with the patient and family is an essential component of health literacy and end-of-life care. Nurses should ask patients about their personal goals of care. This can be accomplished by seeking opportunities to interact and engage the patient and family; doing so builds mutual respect and encourages meaningful feedback from patients and families. Nurses should also explore how the patient and family prefer to make life-altering decisions. Some cultures prefer not to discuss end-of-life care with the patient. It is important to find out if this is the case. Approaching the patient together with family may facilitate a mutually beneficial plan that leads to optimal information sharing (von Gunten et al., 2000).

Step 4:   Deliver the information.

It is important for nurses to speak in plain language using words that are familiar to the patient and family (Sudore & Schillinger, 2009). Speaking slowly, providing the most important information first, allowing the patient and/or family to absorb and process the information before moving on to the next topic is extremely important (von Gunten et al., 2000). During end-of-life conferencing with patients and family members, the nurse should recommend that someone serve as a scribe to record important information that was discussed during the meeting. This will provide a record of important talking points that may assist the patient and/or family in decision making at a future time. Use of illustrations, pictures, scans, and models should also be considered whenever possible to enhance comprehension. The only way to know if the information provided was understood is to use the "teach-back" technique. The nurse might say to a family member after a teaching session, "I have given you a lot of information and I want to be sure I was clear about how your brother should take his pain medication after he is discharged from the hospital. Since you are going to be caring for your brother when he gets home, can you show me how you are going to give him his pain medicine?" (Doak et al., 2007; Paasche-Orlow, Schillinger, Greene, & Wagner, 2006; von Gunten et al., 2000). This technique provides an opportunity for the nurse to assess understanding and provide remediation as needed.

Step 5:   Respond to emotions.

Having critical conversations with patients and families often elicits a number of emotional responses. It is important for the nurse to allow the expression of emotions by listening attentively and quietly. Being aware of nonverbal communication and having the ability to show compassion further strengthen the nurse–patient relationship (von Gunten et al., 2000).

Step 6:   Establish goals of care and treatment priorities.

It is imperative to give patients and families time to absorb and process the critical information that was provided. Nurses need to be mindful not to use words that cause confusion. For example: "It's time to talk about pulling back treatment." This statement may be misconstrued as abandonment (von Gunten et al., 2000, p. 3052). To prevent unintentional consequences, it is vital to use language that emphasizes goals of care (von Gunten et al., 2000). Numerous reasonable goals and treatment options exist in the current heath care arena including curative options, prolongation of life, maintenance of current health status, relief of suffering and issues encompassing quality of life. Implementation of goals of care is not a straightforward process and may apply to specific circumstances throughout the disease trajectory (von Gunten et al., 2000). Empowering patients and families to further develop their health literacy skills can assist them in understanding complex information to gain greater control over their life circumstances (Nutbeam, 2000).

Step 7:   Establish a plan.

It is extremely important to help patients and families to anticipate their experiences within the health care setting (Doak et al., 2007). Providing clear, concise explanations to patients can make their experiences "less traumatic and more manageable" (Doak et al., 2007, p 160). Additional information regarding tests and procedures should be discussed along with the general care plan, symptom management, treatment options, and ongoing emotional support (von Gunten et al., 2000). Providing an orientation is an excellent way to assist patients and families to know what they can expect.

    The orientation should include these five tips:

1. Many patients and families are not prepared to answer questions. It is helpful to tell patients and families that they will be asked many questions by many different health care providers so that patients and families can be prepared in advance. If this information is withheld, the patient and family may perceive the wrong impression that the health care team is not communicating properly (Doak et al., 2007).

2. Tell the patient and family that they will be receiving treatment from many different professionals. Explain scheduling and the different types of health care providers they will encounter. Make certain that patients and families understand that health care professionals share information through the patients' medical record (Doak et al., 2007).

3. Legitimize asking of questions about words that are not understood by the patient. Encourage patients and families to ask questions and request illustrations and or models to further enhance comprehension (Doak et al., 2007).

4. Help patients and families to understand that results from laboratory tests or procedures sometimes take days or longer. Explain that in some cases many different health care professionals have to review the test results (Doak et al., 2007).

5. Help patients to understand the importance of follow-up visits. Explain that visiting their health care professional is important to keep track of how they are doing.

Be sure to utilize health literate reading materials and videos to further enhance communication and comprehension (Doak et al., 2007).

End-of-Life Material

Utilizing End-of-Life Written Materials and Advance Directives

Advance care planning is another way of setting goals for care. Living will, durable power of attorney for health care, and a health care proxy are all forms of advance directives.

The purpose of advance directives is to provide guidance for the type of medical care the patient prefers in the event that he or she is unable make health care decisions (von Gunten et al., 2000). Approximately one third of the adult population has completed an advance directive (Benson & Aldrich, 2012). Despite advance directives being supported by state and federal laws, there are multiple barriers to their completion; lack of education on the part of health care professionals regarding how to approach end-of-life discussions, patients and families' cultural preferences about life-altering and sustaining treatments and poorly written instructions (Benson & Aldrich, 2012). How a person learns about advance directives may also be an important factor in its completion.

The readability of written end-of-life materials and advance directives may also contribute to their underutilization. Many end-of-life documents accessible on the Internet and websites of well-known U.S. Hospice and Palliative Care Organizations far exceed the reading ability of average Americans (Ache & Wallace, 2009). Most materials are written well above the recommended sixth grade level, are text dense, contain too much information, are complicated with medical jargon, and are dependent on words alone (Ache & Wallace, 2009; Sudore & Schillinger, 2009). The consequences of poorly written end-of-life materials present significant barriers to informed decision making and to honoring an individuals' end-of-life choices.

End-of-life patient education materials and advance directives can potentially offer a wealth of knowledge and information to help patients and their loved ones when making life-altering decisions (Ache & Wallace, 2009). It is important for health care professionals to use end-of-life written materials and advance directive documents as a complement to oral communication and educational sessions. This provides an opportunity to address the topic in its situational context, individualize the educational session; encouraging questions and allowing for remediation through the use of teach back. Providing written material as a single entity should be discouraged. Incorporating the tenets of health literacy into both oral and written communication will ensure that patients and their surrogates make informed decisions based on accurate and understandable information (Ache & Wallace, 2009).

Nursing Implications

Understanding the consequences of low health literacy and its impact on chronic disease management and end-of-life care is important to professional nursing. Nurses are at the forefront of patient education and care for diverse populations across the life span in multiple health care environments (American Association of Colleges of Nursing [AACN], 2008). Nurses are expected to provide "appropriate patient teaching that reflects developmental stage, age, culture, spirituality, patient preferences and health literacy considerations to foster patient engagement in their care" (AACN, 2008, p. 31). Nurses serve as patient and surrogate advocates and are responsible to understand and respect the variations and complexities of care and the importance of accessible health resources integral in caring for patients and families (AACN, 2008).

The dynamic arena of health care demands that nurses be well equipped to integrate and apply knowledge that leads to positive patient outcomes. Many nurses do not have adequate education in end-of-life care and are unaware of the impact that low health literacy has on an individual's ability to understand, access, and act upon his or her health information (Cormier & Kotrlik, 2007; Grant et al., 2006; Jukkala, Deupree, & Graham, 2009; Masabasco-O'Connell & Fry-Bowers, 2011; Nielsen-Bohlman, Panzer, & Kindig, 2004; Sand-Jecklin, Murray, Summers, & Watson, 2010; Scheckel, Emery, & Noesek, 2010).

Various approaches to teaching end-of-life care have been identified in the literature. Specialized palliative care educational programs are currently available for physicians and nurses through the Education for Physicians on End-of-Life Care (EPEC) and the End-of-Life Nursing Education Consortium (ELNEC), respectively (Lentz & Sherman, 2006).

The ELNEC was developed and implemented as a national initiative to improve end-of-life care by nurses across all practice settings (Grant et al., 2013). The ELNEC curriculum addresses nurses' personal attitudes, knowledge, and skills in providing of end-of-life care. The nine educational train-the-trainer modules offer an overview of palliative nursing care; pain and symptom management; grief, loss, and bereavement; communication; ethical issues; cultural and spiritual aspects of palliative care; the dying process during the final hours of life; and achieving quality palliative care. The program further stresses the integral role nurses play in helping patients and families identify realistic goals and outcomes of care, use advance directives, access palliative care and hospice as strategies to improve quality of life, and reduce cost (Witt, LaPorte-Matzo, Rogers, McLaughlin, & Virani, 2002). Currently, few data exist to support that palliative and end-of-life nursing education are linked to patient and system outcomes. Evidence continues to grow as new state-funded grant programs are initiated. Collaboration between ELNEC and the Archstone Foundation, the mission of which is to prepare society to care for an aging population, has resulted in educating a number of nurses and other health care professionals as ELNEC trainers (Grant et al., 2013).

The field of health literacy is new and untried. The majority of health care professionals have not been educated in recognizing the impact of low health literacy on effective communication (Coleman, 2011). The literature suggests that workshops be provided to nurse faculty to aid in curricula development and integration of health literacy within the students clinical experiences (Cormier & Kotrlik, 2007; Scheckel et al., 2010). However, barriers to health literacy education are prevalent and competencies remain undefined (Coleman, 2011).

The ELNEC model may serve as a paradigm to integrate health literacy into nursing education.

References

Ache, K. A., & Wallace, L. S. (2009). Are end of life patient education materials readable? *Palliative Medicine, 23*, 545–548.

American Association of Colleges of Nursing. (2008). *The essentials of baccalaureate education for professional nursing practice.* Retrieved from http://www.aacn.nche .edu/education-resources/baccessentials08.pdf

Angus, D. E., Barnato, A., Linde-Zwirble, W. T., Weissfeld, L. A., Watson, R. S., Rickert, T., & Rubenfeld, G. D. (2004). Use of intensive care as the end of life in the United States: An epidemiologic study. *Critical Care Medicine, 32*, 638–643.

Benson, W. F., & Aldrich, N. (2012). *Advance care planning: Ensuring your wishes are known and honored if you are unable to speak for yourself* (Critical issue brief, Centers for Disease Control and Prevention). Retrieved from http://www.cdc.gov/aging

Billings, J. A., & Block, S. (1997). Palliative care in undergraduate medical education: Status report and future directions. *Journal of the American Medical Association, 278*(9), 733–738.

Center to Advance Palliative Care. (2011). *Public opinion research on palliative care.* Retrieved from http://www.capc.org/tools-for-palliative-care-programs/ marketing/public-opinion-research/2011-public-opinion-research-on- palliative-care.pdf

Coleman, C. (2011). Teaching health care professionals about health literacy: A review of the literature. *Nursing Outlook, 59*, 70–78. doi:10.1016/j .outlook.2010.12.004

Cormier, C., & Kotrlik, J. W. (2007). Health literacy knowledge and experience of senior baccalaureate nursing students. *Journal of Nursing Education, 48*(5), 237–247. doi:10.9999

DeSpelder, L. A., & Strickland, A. L. (2010). *The last dance: Encountering death and dying* (9th ed.). New York, NY: McGraw Hill.

DeWalt, D. A. (2007). Low health literacy: Epidemiology and interventions. *North Carolina Medical Journal, 68*(5), 327–330.

Doak, C. C., Doak, L. G., & Root, J. H. (2007). Tips on teaching. In C. C. Doak, L. G. Doak, & J. H. Root, *Teaching patients with low literacy skills.* (2nd ed., pp. 151–166). Philadelphia, PA: Lippincott.

Edwards, M., Wood, F., Davies, M., & Edwards, A. (2012). The development of health literacy in patients with a long-term health condition: The health literacy pathway model. *BMC Public Health, 12*(130). Retrieved from http//www .biomedcentral.com/1471-2458/12/130

Fisher, S. M., Gozansky, W. S., Kutner, J. S., Chomiak, A., & Kramer, A. (2003). Palliative care education: An intervention to improve residents' knowledge and attitudes. *Journal of Palliative Medicine, 6*(3), 391–397.

Fraser, H. C., Kutner, J. S., & Pfeifer, M. P. (2001). Senior medical students' perceptions of adequacy of education on end of life issues. *Journal of Palliative Medicine, 4,* 337–343.

Goodman, D. C., Esty, A. R., Fischer, E. S., & Chiang, C. H. (2011). *Trends and variations in end-of-life care for Medicare beneficiaries with severe chronic illness* (Report of the Dartmouth Atlas Project). Retrieved from http://www .dartmouthatlas.org/downloads/reports/EOL_Trend_Report_0411.pd

Goodman, D. C., Morden, N. E., Chiang, C. H., Fisher, E. S., & Wennberg, J. E. (2013). *Trends in cancer care near the end of life* (Report of the Dartmouth Atlas Project). Retrieved from http://www.rwjf.org/en/research-publications/ find-rwjf-research/2013/09/trends-in-cancer

Grant, M., Wiencek, C., Virani, R., Uman, G., Munevar, C., Malloy, P., & Ferrell, B. (2013). End of life education in acute and critical care: The California ELNEC project. *American Association of Critical Care Nurse Advanced Critical Care, 2,* 121–129. doi:10.1097/NCI.0b013e3182832a94

Institute of Medicine. (1997). Summary. In M. J. Field & C. K. Cassel (Eds.), *Approaching death: Improving care at the end of life* (pp 1–33.). Washington, DC: The National Academies Press.

Institute of Medicine. (2001). Background and recommendations. In K. M. Foley & H. Gelband (Eds.), *Improving palliative care for cancer care* (pp. 9–64). Washington, DC: The National Academies Press.

Institute of Medicine. (2002). Introduction. In M. J. Field & R. E. Behrman (Eds.), *When children die: Improving palliative and end-of-life care for children and their families* (pp. 19–40). Washington, DC: The National Academies Press.

Jukkala, A., Deupree, J. P., & Graham, S. (2009). Knowledge of limited literacy in an academic health center. *Journal of Continuing Education in Nursing, 40*(7), 298–302.

Kelly, P. A., & Haidet, P. (2006). Physician overestimation of patient literacy: A potential source of health care disparities. *Patient Education and Counseling, 66*(2007), 119–122 . doi:10.1016/j.pec.2006.10.007

Koh, H. K., Berwick, D. M., Clancey, C. M., Baur, C., Harris, L. M., & Zerhusen, E. G. (2012). New federal policy initiatives to boost health literacy can help improve the nations move beyond the cycle of costly crisis care. *Health Affairs, 31*(2), 434–443. Retrieved from http//www.content .healthaffairs.org.doi:10.1377/hlthaff.2011.1169

Kung, H. C., Hoyert, D. L., Xu, J. Q., & Murphy, S. L. (2008). Deaths: Final data for 2005. *National Vital Statistics Reports, 5*(10). Retrieved from http://www.cdc.gov/nchs/data/nvsr/nvsr56/nvsr56_10.pdf

Kutner, M., Greenberg, E., Jin, Y., & Paulsen, C. (2006). *The health literacy of American adults: Results from the 2003 National Assessment of Adult Literacy* (NCES 2006-483). U.S. Department of Education. Washington, DC: National Center for Education Statistics.

Lentz, J., & Sherman, D. (2006). Professional organizations and certifications in hospice and palliative care. In M. LaPorte & D. Witt Sherman, *Palliative care nursing* (2nd ed., pp. 117–130). New York, NY: Springer Publishing Company.

Levin, T. T., Moreno, B., Silvester, W., & Kissane, D. W. (2010). End of life communication in the intensive care unit. *General Hospital Psychiatry, 32*, 433–442. doi:10.1016/jgenhosppsych.2010.04.007

Lynn, J. (2000). Learning to care for people with chronic illness facing the end of life [Editorial]. *Journal of the American Medical Association, 284*(19), 2508–2511.

Masabasco-O'Connell, A., & Fry-Bowers, E. K. (2011). Knowledge and perception of health literacy among nursing professionals. *Journal of Health Communication, 16*, 295–304. doi:10.1080/10810730.2011.604389

McKinney, M. (2010). Where you live = how you die. *Modern Healthcare, 40*(47), 6–8.

Meier, D. (2013, April). Palliative care 2020: Matching care to patient and family needs. In C. Davis, K. Gottlieb, K. Robinson, & S. S. Stout (Co-chairs), *14th Annual International Summit on Improving Patient Care in the Office Practice and the Community.* Symposium conducted at the meeting of The Institute for Healthcare Improvement, Scottsdale, AZ.

Morita, T., Miyashita, M., Tsuneto, S., Sato, K., & Shima, Y. (2009). Late referrals to palliative care units in Japan: Nationwide follow-up survey and effects of palliative care team involvement after the Cancer Control Act. *Journal of Pain and Symptom Management, 38*, 191–196.

National Hospice and Palliative Care Organization. (2012). *Facts and figures: Hospice care in America.* Retrieved from http://www.nhpco.org/sites/default/files/public/Statistics_Research/2012_Facts_Figures.pdf

National Hospice and Palliative Care Organization. (2013). *History of hospice: A historical perspective.* Retrieved from http://www.nhpco.org/history-hospice-care

Nielsen-Bohlman, L., Panzer, A. M., & Kindig, D. A. (2004). *Health literacy: A prescription to end the confusion.* Washington DC: The National Academies Press.

Nutbeam, D. (2000). Health literacy as a public goal: A challenge for contemporary health education and communication strategies into the 21st century. *Health Promotion International, 15*(3), 259–267.

Nutbeam, D. (2008). The evolving concept of health literacy. *Social, Science and Medicine. 67,* 2072–2078. doi:10.1016/j.socsimed.2008.09.050

Paasche-Orlow, M. K., Schillinger, D., Greene, S. M., & Wagner, E. H. (2006). How health care systems can begin to address the challenges of limited literacy. *Journal of General Internal Medicine,* 21, 884–887. doi:10.1111/j .1525-1497.2006.00544.x

Peters, L., Cant, R., Payne, S., O'Connor, M., McDermott, F., Hood, K., ... Shimoinaba, K. (2013). How death anxiety impacts nurses caring for patients at the end of life: A review of the literature. *The Open Nursing Journal, 7,* 12–24.

Sand-Jecklin, K., Murray, B., Summers, B., & Watson, J. (2010). Educating nursing students about health literacy: From the classroom to the patient bedside. *The Online Journal of Issues in Nursing, 15*(3). Retrieved from http:// www.nursingworld.org/MainMenuCategories/ANAMarketplace/ ANAPeriodicals/OJINTable

Savory, E. A., & Marco, C. A. (2009). End of life issues in the acute and critically ill patient. *Scandinavian Journal of Trauma Resuscitation and Emergency Medicine, 17*(21). Retrieved from www.sjtrem.com/content/17/1/21.doi: 10.1186/1757-7241-17-21

Scheckel, M., Emery, N., & Noesek, C. (2010). Addressing health literacy: The experience of undergraduate nursing students. *Journal of Clinical Nursing, 19,* 794–802. doi:101111/j.1365-27.02.2009.022991.x

Speros, C. (2005). Health literacy: Concept analysis. *Journal of Advanced Nursing, 50,* 633–640. doi:10.1111/j.1365-2648.2005.03448.x

Sudore, R. L., & Schillinger, D. (2009). Interventions to improve care for patients with limited literacy. *Journal of Clinical Outcomes Management, 16*(1), 20–29.

SUPPORT Investigators. (1995). Controlled trial to improve care for seriously ill hospitalized patients. *Journal of American Medical Association, 274*(20), 1591–1598.

Temel, J., Greer, J. A., Muzikansky, M. A., Gallagher, E. R., Admane, S., Jackson, V. A., ... Lynch, T. J. (2010). Early palliative care for patients with metastatic non-small cell lung cancer. *New England Journal of Medicine, 363,* 733–742.

The Dartmouth Atlas of Health Care. (2013). *End of life care.* Retrieved from http://www.dartmouthatlas.org/keyissues/issue.aspx?con=2944

The Joint Commission. (2010). *Advancing effective communication, cultural competence and patient and family-centered care: A roadmap for hospitals.* Oak-brook Terrace, IL: Author.

Thorpe, K. E., Ogden, L. L., & Galactionova, K. (2010). Chronic conditions account for rise in Medicare spending from 1987-2006. *Health Affairs, 29*(4), 718–724.

von Gunten, C. F., Ferris, F. D., & Emmanuel, L. L. (2000). Ensuring competency in end of life care. *Journal of the American Medical Association, 284*(23), 3051–3057.

Wennberg, J. E., Fisher, E. S., Goodman, D. C., & Skinner, J. S. (2008). *Tracking the care of patients with severe chronic illness. The Dartmouth Atlas of Health Care.* Retrieved from http://www.dartmouth.ed~jskinner/documents/2008_Chronic_Care_Atlas.pdf

Wennberg, J. E., Fisher, E. S., Skinner, J. S., & Bronner, K. K. (2007). Extending the P4P agenda, part 2: How Medicare can reduce waste and improve care for the chronically ill. *Health Affairs, 26*(6), 1575–1585.

Witt-Sherman, D., LaPorte-Matzo, M., Rogers, S., McLaughlin, M., & Virani, R. (2002). Achieving quality care at the end of life: A focus of the End-of-Life Nursing Education Consortium (ELNEC) curriculum. *Journal of Professional Nursing, 18*(5), 255–262.

World Health Organization. (2013). *WHO definition of palliative care.* Retrieved from http://www.who.int/cancer/palliative/definition/en

Wright, A. A., Keating, N. L., Balboni, T. A., Mantulonis, U. A., Block, S., & Prigerson, H. G. (2010). Place of death: Correlations with quality of life patients with cancer and predictors of bereaved caregivers' mental health. *Journal of Clinical Oncology, 28*(29), 4457–4464.

Pediatrics

Gloria M. Collura
Suzanne Monteleone

The single biggest problem in communication is the illusion that it has taken place.

—George Bernard Shaw

Case Scenario

The neonatal intensive care unit was discharging a premature infant born at 24 weeks that was now 36 weeks of age. The infant had a hospital course complicated by sepsis and bronchopulmonary dysplasia. The infant was discharged on multiple medications including ferrous sulfate and would require follow-up care. On the day of discharge the parents were provided education on medications and administration, utilizing the medications the hospital had provided as an inpatient to demonstrate administration. The prescriptions were provided to the parents and they were instructed to pick them up from the pharmacy as soon as possible to begin administration with the next required dose. The parents filled the prescriptions and were administering the medications as they had been taught. The infant had a scheduled visit with the prenatal clinic 1 week postdischarge. At this visit it was discovered the infant had been receiving 10 times the dose of ferrous sulfate each day that week and was suffering from constipation.

221

Several factors may have led to this significant outcome. The parents were taught how to administer the medication in the hospital before discharge but when it was demonstrated, it was done using a different measuring appliance than what came with the prescription from the pharmacy. The pharmacy supplied a different concentration of the liquid, which the parents did not realize. Neither the nurses nor the clinical pharmacists incorporated teach-back or show-me after they demonstrated the administration of ferrous sulfate. There were no follow-up phone calls to assess and reinforce teaching if needed.

Current Issues in Pediatric Health Literacy

Although low health literacy has been viewed as a major public health issue, the vital issue of low health literacy and the specific implications and relevance to the care of children and families remain opportunities for ongoing research. To date, the targeted populations in research efforts to understand and enhance low health literacy have been primarily adults. The goals for children and their adult caregivers remain similar: to enhance the health care system, increase access and inclusion, decrease disparities, and ultimately improve overall health outcomes (Abrams, Klass, & Dreyer, 2009, p. S262).

The areas of uniqueness and complexity when addressing pediatric health literacy are that the health literacy skills of the child, as well as the parents, family members, or caregivers, must be considered. In addition, a young child's health literacy will continue to evolve as the child grows, learns over time, and matures (Abrams et al., 2009). Health literacy research data of young children are difficult to report, however, "about 1 in 3 children are identified by state and national tests as reading below their grade level" (National Center for Education Statistics, 2005). In addition, similar to many other health care professionals, it has been suggested that pediatric providers overestimate the health literacy levels of the families of the children they care for (Wittich, Mangan, Grad, Wand, & Gerald, 2007). Unfortunately, another similarity to the adult counterparts is that most child health information is written well above the eighth-grade reading level, making it difficult for parents and caregivers to understand (Doak, Doak, & Root, 1996).

In addition to the general research on health literacy that can be applied to parents and caregivers, the American Academy of Pediatrics (AAP) has been a very active partner in addressing the health literacy issues that are more uniquely related to parent and caregiver understanding. In November 2008, a conference was convened on health literacy and pediatrics called "A Health-Literate America: Where Do Children Fit In?" The purpose of the conference was to examine health literacy–related gaps and opportunities specifically in regard to children and children's health. *Plain Language Pediatrics: Health Literacy Strategies and Communication Resources for Common Pediatric Topics* was published by the AAP to enhance plain language communication in the pediatric office setting and offers plain language educational materials in English and Spanish as reproducible resources for pediatricians. The AAP has developed webinars and continuing medical education courses as vehicles to enhance awareness, knowledge, understanding, and implications specific to pediatric health literacy.

Significance of Health Literacy and Children's Health

In the United States, there are approximately 74 million children under the age of 18, representing approximately 24% of the total population. The population under the age of 18 grew at a rate of 2.6% between 2000 and 2010 (U.S. Census, 2010).

Medication Use in Children

In 2011, "10 million children in the United States had a health problem for which prescription medication had been taken regularly for at least 3 months (14%). Eighteen percent of youths aged 12 to 17 were on regular medication compared with 13% of children aged 5 to 11 and 9% of children aged 4 and under. Children with a parent who had an education beyond a high school diploma were more likely to have been on regular medication (15%) than children whose parent did not obtain a high school diploma or the equivalent (9%)" (Bloom, Cohen, & Freeman, 2012).

Health Status

When reviewing the data for children's health status, the majority of U.S. children are fortunate to have excellent health (42 million or 56%), and another 20 million children have very good health (27%) (Bloom et al., 2012). Interestingly, as the level of education increased for the parents, the excellent health status of the children also increased. This is further illustrated by the reported data associated with children's health; 43% of children in poor families were in excellent health compared with 64% of children in families that were not poor (Bloom et al., 2012). Health status disparities between private and public health coverage were reported; "Children with private health insurance were more likely to be in excellent health (64%) than children with Medicaid or other public coverage (46%)" (Bloom et al., 2012).

Contact With Health Care Professionals

The "majority of children (75%) had contact with a physician or other health care professional at some point in the past 6 months, although children with a parent that was educated beyond high school were more likely to have had contact with a health care professional in the past 6 months than those who had less than a high school education" (Bloom et al., 2012). In 2011, over 9 million U.S. children had an emergency department visit in the past year, while 4.3 million had two or more visits (Bloom et al., 2012).

Health Insurance Coverage

In 2011, 5 million children had no health insurance coverage and "Hispanic children (13%) were at least twice as likely as non-Hispanic White (5%) and Black (6%) children to be uninsured for health care"(Bloom et al., 2012). Income was also associated with health insurance as families with an income of less than $35,000 to $49,999 had an increased likelihood (10%–11%) of not having insurance as those families with an income of $100,000 or more (2%) (Bloom et al., 2012). In addition, children living in single father family homes were more likely to be uninsured for health care than children in two parent families or single mother family homes.

As illustrated by the above data, significant areas of risk from low health literacy in the pediatric population are general health status, access to health care, medication use and safety, and visits to health care professionals. Having access to pediatric primary care is the first step in health promotion and increasing health literacy in the parent and child. Children of caregivers with low health literacy have the disadvantages of not having direct access to primary care and an increase in potential health care needs not being addressed (Sanders, Thompson, & Wilkinson, 2007).

Another area of risk is harm due to medication errors from misinterpretation of dosing charts, correlating to low numeracy skills (Lokker et al., 2009).

Poor childhood nutrition is associated with low literacy skills, with caregivers being less likely to look at nutrition labels on food products. It is also indicated that parents with poor health literacy were not likely to have an accurate perception of their child's weight (Rothman et al., 2006). Some studies suggest mothers with low health literacy skills are more likely to smoke, therefore exposing the child to secondhand smoke in the environment (Fredrickson et al., 1995).

Health Literacy of Parent or Caregiver: Infants and Young Children

Pediatric health literacy is unique in that it begins with the parents or caregivers own health literacy while acting as the surrogate for the child; over time, as the child matures, the child begins to play a larger role in his or her own health and well-being (Borzekowski, 2009). Many caregivers of young children do not have adequate literacy skills to understand and follow child preventive health messages. More than one in three young adults of child-bearing age have limited health literacy (Sanders, Federico, Klass, Abrams, & Dreyer, 2009) and children of parents with low health literacy are at risk for having unmet health care needs (Yin et al., 2009). Additional findings have shown that 36% of the population is not able to perform basic child preventive health tasks such as using an immunization schedule, following recommendations from a preventive health brochure, and interpreting a growth chart (Kutner, Greenberg, Jin, & Paulsen, 2006). Research has demonstrated "lesser command of the English language was associated with poorer child health status" and children of limited English proficient parents were three times as likely to have spent at least 1 sick day in bed over the previous year (Monsen, 2007).

There is a strong motivation among pediatricians to encourage even young children to become knowledgeable regarding health care and opportunities to improve their own health. For this to occur it is important to begin to develop a child's literacy of health at a young age, taking into consideration the child's stage of development. For preschool children, using a recognizable storyline to create a television program aimed at reducing injury is a simple way to begin to make them aware of their surroundings and potential areas for injury (Borzekowski, 2009).

Caregivers may choose to limit children's exposure to health-related issues in an attempt to protect them; often, selection of treatments, procedures, and surgeries is done without children being present. However inclusion in this process can empower children and educate them to health issues affecting them, in turn allowing them to be a part of their own health and assist with improving it. With children becoming active participants in their health, they are more apt to build on health-promoting activities, since perceptions of health and behaviors formed during childhood have an impact on adult health patterns (Roter, 2000).

It is a necessity for parents and caregivers to have the skills to ensure their children will receive adequate health care. These skills include obtaining health insurance as well as reading medication and nutrition labels. Unfortunately a national study examined health literacy among a population of parents in the United States and revealed one in four parents have limited health literacy skills. In the current state of child health-related issues, there are increased demands for parents to have a higher literacy skill to comprehend and protect their child from harm (Yin et al., 2009). Study results indicated there are areas for improvement in regard to medication administration in the pediatric outpatient area. The inability to interpret medication labels was identified as an area of risk for both the adult and pediatric populations.

These study results have identified the role of the parents' health literacy and the health outcomes for their child. There is a large number of parents in the United States lacking health literacy skills; this will affect the health outcomes of their children (Yin et al., 2009). In examining the literacy skills of parents it is evident that children of parents with higher literacy skills are more likely to have better health outcomes in relation to sexually transmitted diseases, obesity, and substance abuse (Sanders et al., 2009).

Understanding the significant issue of low health literacy among parents/caregivers, the following interventions were developed based on the 2004 Institute of Medicine report. These interventions are based on individualized patient care and the care received from a health care system, the educational system, and the community (Sanders, Shaw, Guez, Baur, & Rudd, 2009).

Adolescent Health Literacy

Adolescents are at a crucial stage of development, learning skills they will carry into adulthood. Prevention of low literacy is the key to assisting a child with being able to form health literacy skills for later in life. As adolescents increasingly become more involved in their own health care, a specific focus on health literacy is needed (Manganello, 2007).

Health literacy is crucial for the adolescent suffering from a chronic illness such as cystic fibrosis, asthma, diabetes, and mental illness. As a result of having a chronic illness, these adolescents will have more interactions with the health care system than an adolescent who is not suffering from a chronic illness. The goal is to have the adolescent participate in his or her care to the fullest extent possible, which requires health literacy skills (Boice, 1998). It is common for many adolescents to rely on the Internet as source of information for health-related issues, indicating the need for them to be taught how to differentiate reliable from unreliable sources. In addition, the adolescent is receiving large quantities of information from the school and it is imperative this information be understood by the adolescent (Raver, Hancock, Ingersoll, & 2004). The framework for adolescent health literacy examines how individual characteristics, peer–parent influences, and health care educational systems all combine to influence one's health literacy.

Media is another important component of and powerful influence on this framework, as it is such a large part of an adolescent's daily life. It is also a large source of health information for the adolescent (Nielsen-Bohlman, Panzer, & Kindig, 2004). Peer and parent influences are important in this framework as well. Parent health literacy can impact health outcomes for the adolescent. As previously mentioned in this chapter, parents' health literacy can directly affect health outcomes for their children (Yin et al., 2009), as parents are a major component in developing the health literacy of their children. Peer groups play a large role in the life of the adolescent and therefore can greatly influence the adolescent in matters of health behaviors (Nielsen-Bohlman et al., 2004). Both education and health care systems can largely impact the adolescent lifestyle and can be used as vehicles to promote health literacy and health promotion.

The impact of the education system is significant and its role in health literacy should not be taken lightly. The adolescent continues to cognitively and socially develop and many opportunities exist for the education system to develop and enhance skills specific to health literacy. Teachers can play a vital role in educating the adolescent on how to comprehend and evaluate health information. To do this effectively, teachers should receive regular continuing development in this area (Nielsen-Bohlman et al., 2004).

The health system is an additional component in this framework, as it is a vehicle that can impact access to health care, and the way health care information is communicated to the adolescent and family. This communication can be oral, from provider to adolescent, or via written materials such as brochures and pamphlets. Ensuring that both written communication and oral communication are at the health literacy level of the adolescent is crucial in developing these skills for the adolescent (Nielsen-Bohlman et al., 2004).

Research must continue in the area of adolescent health literacy. Areas to be addressed are developing and validating tools to measure health literacy in the adolescent population, examining predictors of health literacy levels among adolescents and the relationship to health outcomes, and lastly developing and evaluating interventions that can promote a greater understanding of health information for adolescents (Manganello, 2007).

Enhancing Child and Parent Health Literacy

Individualized Patient Care

The child and parent are entitled to receive clear information pertaining to the health risks and issues associated with childhood including but not limited to immunizations, injury prevention, and nutrition. To accomplish this goal all members of the primary care team should receive education on how to communicate effectively. This should include use of teach-back and allowing the parent, child, or caregiver to participate in the decision-making processes (Flowers, 2006). Providers should understand the importance of including the child's grade level in their assessment, to identify issues early, and to provide age-appropriate information on interventions. The office setting is a wonderful opportunity to provide education to parents and children, utilizing easy-to-read print as well as audiovisual tools to reinforce preventive health (Wolff et al., 2009). Pediatric nurses are involved in both parent and child education on a regular basis and can be role models for all members of the health care team or office practice setting. As pediatric nurses are well aware, the use of credible, culturally appropriate written materials is vital to support and enhance the health information provided to the child and parent. Videos and other nonprint resources can be utilized as communication tools in specific situations such as the demonstration of proper dental care or handwashing (Sanders et al., 2009).

The Health Care System

The complex environment of the health care system can be overwhelming to the parent and child with low health literacy. In addition, parents with limited English proficiency were significantly more likely to have barriers when accessing health care (Monsen, 2007). As families and caregivers of pediatric patients try to navigate complex health care systems, it is imperative that nurses work toward meeting the health literacy needs of families and pediatric patients. This must be done so caregivers can make the best health decisions for their child.

Health care systems have been defined as the "complete network of agencies, facilities, and all providers of health care in a specified geographic area. Nursing services are integral to all levels and patterns of care and nurses form the largest number of providers in a health care system" (Elsevier, 2009).

The health system has a direct impact upon how accessible health care is and how effectively health information is communicated to the child and parent (Nielsen-Bohlman et al., 2004). All health information should be tailored to the child's needs and developmental stage, and access to low literacy health information with standardized information should be available to both the parent and child. Ongoing monitoring of health literacy–related metrics should be included in measures of quality (Sanders et al., 2009) as these are directly related to patient outcomes, patient safety, and patient satisfaction.

The Educational System

The educational system provides an excellent opportunity to build health literacy skills. The collaboration of child health researchers, health care professionals, and educators can help to create curricula to guide building health literacy skills from kindergarten through grade 12. Classrooms should be used to reinforce information about individual health behaviors. Together, efforts can reinforce health promotion and truly integrate health-related activities with the lessons being taught (see Chapter 2, "Low Health Literacy and Implications," p. 45). These efforts should be modeled on evidence-based campaigns to promote adolescent health, such as antidrug, anti alcohol, and anti tobacco campaigns (Sanders et al., 2009).

Community Partners

Community settings should focus on child health promotion messaging and events to promote child health. Communities offering fairs that provide education to parents and children regarding healthy eating, injury prevention, helmet fittings, and child passenger safety can improve child health outcomes (Sanders et al., 2009).

Pediatricians and Health Literacy

Recently, health literacy is viewed as a partnership between the health care professional and the person receiving the care. Health literacy should incorporate the skills, or lack thereof, of the health care professional as well. The pediatrician plays a vital role in the area of health literacy and can participate in the process to lessen the gap that exists between the health literacy skills of the children and parents and the information being provided.

A national survey done by the AAP between March and August of 2007 reported 81% of pediatricians indicated they were aware that a caregiver had not understood the necessary medical information provided and 44% were aware of an error in patient care due to health literacy issues (Turner et al., 2009). The survey was developed to assess experiences surrounding health literacy and patient communication. Most pediatricians reported using basic communication techniques and were much less likely to use enhanced communication techniques. More than half of the pediatricians agree with the statement "there is not enough time in a pediatric visit to use special communication techniques." Pediatricians surveyed also indicated they were not completely comfortable with their health literacy skills and would take part in education to improve those skills (Turner et al., 2009). This survey has demonstrated the need for further education and implementation of effective communication skills with caregivers and children with low health literacy. Identified barriers included time, access to educational materials, as well as their own limited knowledge of health literacy. Nearly all of the pediatricians that participated in the survey agreed with general health literacy principles such as: improved communication can enhance patient and parent satisfaction; low health literacy skills can lead to errors; enhancing health literacy skills can improve the quality of pediatric health care; and pediatricians can implement strategies to enhance understanding. Although aware of the above principles, there was a common theme of "not having enough time in a pediatric visit" (Turner et al., 2009). In addition, there is a further need to put an action plan in place for interventions to decrease untoward events to the patient as it relates to low health literacy.

Pediatricians can perform a more dynamic assessment, taking note of how the child follows his or her prescribed medical treatment with the parent's assistance. This will assist in determining what role the child should have in self-management of his or her own health and illness in the child's home environment (Borzekowski, 2009).

As communication technologies have expanded over the recent years, and the use and availability of cell phones has increased, a possible strategy to investigate is the use of text messaging reminders, especially for hard-to-reach populations or for complicated scheduling such as immunization compliance (Vilella et al., 2004). Parents may benefit from reminders after an office visit and pediatricians may benefit from additional effective health literacy strategies. Recent studies have suggested that children receive only half of the indicated preventive, acute, or chronic care (Rothman et al., 2009, p. S315). Additional areas of research are needed especially in the area of pediatrics and the unique issues relative to children's health—developmental change of children over time, dependency on parents, differential epidemiology of child health, and different demographic patterns of children and their families (Rothman et al., 2009, p. S315).

Implications to Pediatric Nursing Practice

Health literacy has specific implications to nursing practice in the pediatric population. This can be subdivided into the following categories by type of care delivery as well as the stages of growth and development such as infant–toddler, preschool, school age, and adolescent.

Type of care delivery:

- Inpatient
- Outpatient or ambulatory care

Inpatient Setting

Oftentimes, when a child and parent or caregiver enter the hospital for the first time, there is a level of anxiety, nervousness, and fear of the unknown often due in part to the limited knowledge of the practices and processes in a hospital setting. Perhaps this is the way you felt when you had your first clinical experience as a student nurse.

All parents want to protect their child and there is a feeling of loss of control in the health care setting. This may be a feeling similar to when you sent your child off to school for the first time and anxiously followed the bus, making sure your child got into the classroom safely. Then you may have found yourself sitting at home and wondering if your child was okay. Does he or she know how to get help if needed? Will he or she eat lunch? Unfortunately, there are times when the child is in pain or is confronting a serious illness. This, of course, alters the health literacy skills of both the child and parent or caregiver.

The importance of assessing the health literacy skills from the time families enter the hospital in crucial for nurses. The first interview often sets the tone for the entire inpatient hospital stay and can ultimately affect the outcome for the child. Nurses can learn valuable information that can be helpful when communicating with patients and their families. The below information can help pediatric nurses to individualize their teaching to effectively meet the needs of the child and parent:

- Race, ethnicity, and preferred language to discuss health care
- Educational level of the person receiving the information
- Cultural, religious, and spiritual preferences
- The primary caregiver of the child

This information is invaluable when providing patient-centered individualized care for the child and family. Family-centered care is crucial for obtaining quality outcomes in the pediatric population. The nurses must ensure that the family is engaged, involved, and truly understands all treatment and discharge instructions. For example, when caring for an asthmatic toddler to school-age child, it is necessary to ensure that the family is educated on the triggers of asthma, what triggers are, how to avoid them, and when to start using the inhalers or nebulizer treatments. Incorporating plain language and the teach-back method is essential to ensure understanding is vital. Requesting a home care visit to perform a home assessment may even be necessary, and can assist in reviewing discharge instructions, enhance outcomes, and ultimately avoid unnecessary readmissions.

When a child and family's preferred language is other than English, utilizing qualified interpretation services to teach the child and family and provide written instructions translated into their preferred language will assist in treatment adherence and compliance.

Another challenging example is adolescent patients with juvenile diabetes. Without proper compliance with diet, use of insulin, and monitoring of glucose levels, these children will unfortunately experience increased readmissions. More importantly, an inability to follow through with prescribed treatment can lead to further poor outcomes ranging from heart disease to diabetic coma and even death. This specific pediatric patient population needs to have critical literacy skills, which can be defined as "the ability to critically analyze information and use this information to exert greater control over life events and situation" (Nutbeam, 2000). Assessing the health literacy skills of the adolescent is important for nurses to incorporate into their patient assessment. There are a limited number of tools available to measure health literacy and most are geared to the adult population. Recently, an adolescent version of The Rapid Estimate of Adult Literacy in Medicine (REALM) was developed called the REALM-Teen. This version is similar to the REALM format but uses terminology more familiar to teens (Davis et al., 2006).

Outpatient or Ambulatory Setting

This category refers to the pediatric patients that have any type of ambulatory or outpatient procedures and care that do not require an inpatient hospital stay. Examples include ambulatory surgery, outpatient MRI, CAT scans, x-rays, or clinic care for more chronic conditions. The ambulatory setting provides many opportunities for pediatric nurses to enhance their ability to quickly assess a child's and the parents' health literacy skills.

Oftentimes, general anesthesia may be needed for an outpatient procedure or surgery in the ambulatory setting. Preparation for the anesthesia includes education and written information at the time of scheduling and reinforcement and review via phone call the night before to ensure nothing-by-mouth guidelines are maintained. Utilizing informational scripts that can be individualized, as well as checklists to standardize the information patients receive, can assist in enhancing effective communication. Continuing to assess and reassess the tools utilized and updating them to meet the needs of this ever-changing population is important as health care is always changing and evolving based on evidence-based practices. Exposure to Child Life Specialists should be mandatory for all pediatric patients undergoing surgery or any procedure. Emergency departments have partnered with Child Life Specialists to distract and decrease anxiety of patients having x-rays, CAT scans, and blood tests. Use of picture books and other props to introduce new concepts to the child and family is an excellent method to decrease stress and increase compliance for the child and family.

The utilization of written materials that are at the proper reading level, are culturally appropriate, inviting, and easy to read and understand can also improve understanding and compliance for some families and patients. Adolescents in particular are very concerned about how they are perceived and are sometimes afraid to ask questions. Having common questions in written material or available as an application for an iPad or smart phone could fit with an adolescent's preferred way to learn and help to promote better understanding and improve compliance for this particular patient population.

Pediatric Nursing Implications

Limited health literacy affects children of all races, income, ages, and education levels. However, the impact of limited health literacy affects lower socioeconomic and minority groups at a disproportional rate. Health literacy affects a person's ability to search for and use health information, adopt healthy behaviors, and act on important health issues. Limited health literacy is also associated with poor health outcomes and higher costs overall (Sanders et al., 2009). This has definite implications to pediatric nursing practice.

One can see from the definition of health care systems that nurses are a major part of the health care experience for the pediatric patient, his or her family, and caregivers. Nurses must lead the way in closing the gap in health literacy in order to ensure the quality and safety of the children we care for. Studies have shown that "1 in 3 American adults has limited health literacy" (Sanders et al., 2009). We must treat the need for health literacy reform in the pediatric population as aggressively as we look for treatments and cures for cancer, diabetes, and heart disease. When parents and caregivers do not understand the instructions and information provided to them, the consequences can be detrimental to the pediatric patient's health outcome and overall quality of life.

Preventive care is ensuring that there is an understanding of the medical recommendations and information related to health services by the patient and, in the case of our younger pediatric patients—infants, toddlers, and preschoolers—by the parent or caregiver. The nurse is primarily the health care professional that ensures this is adequately done.

Pediatric Written Materials

Currently, across the country, information is written anywhere from a fifth-grade reading level up to greater than a 10th-grade reading level. Examples include the Centers for Disease Control and Prevention's polio vaccine information pamphlet, which is at a fifth-grade reading level. There are 26 states that have enrollment forms for the State Children's Health Insurance Program that are written well above the 10th-grade reading level (Sanders et al., 2009). These disparities in readability and understandability of information we provide to our families is a safety issue for our pediatric population. The health care delivery systems in our country must work together to provide opportunities to close the gap in how we provide medical information, medication management, discharge instructions, and other health information to the community. Nurses must be at the forefront of this effort as this has daily implications to their practice.

Fortunately, there have been improvements. Free language interpreter services via phone, video, or on-site persons are assisting nurses and physicians in communicating effectively to obtain medical authorization and consents from our families. In addition, the implementation of vital documents in the preferred languages of the communities served also enhance communication. In these communities, it is even more imperative we improve the health literacy in the written instructions and informational pamphlets given to our pediatric families. We must be sure to obtain guidance from representatives from the communities we serve as we continue to provide culturally and linguistically relevant information. This engagement will help ensure we meet the cultural and linguistic needs of the community and is imperative to success.

Medication Management

Medication errors have received national attention since the release of the Institute of Medicine report *To Err Is Human: Building a Safer Health System*. This has major implications for all pediatric patients but especially those in the outpatient setting and those that are managing chronic illnesses. There is growing acknowledgment that medications are utilized more frequently now in outpatient settings and managed by parents and other lay caregivers. The potential exposure of children to these errors increases with the outpatient settings prescribing more medications, especially to chronically ill children. More than a half million medication errors take place in the outpatient areas every year. With the increase in the number of chronically ill children, medication errors may worsen. A recent study revealed that 70% of preventable adverse drug errors were due to errors in mediation administration, which highlights the important role that health literacy can play in appropriate medication management outside of the hospital setting (Rothman et al., 2009). Nurses play a major role in enhancing the patient's and parents' understanding of medication management, and need to have the skills to assess the health literacy level of the patient and family to ensure the safety of the pediatric patient.

Nursing Implications and Future Recommendations

"Addressing health literacy should be part of the framework for effectively improving delivery of quality child health services" (Abrams, Klass, & Dreyer, 2009, p. S329). As we continue along the path to improving health literacy in our country, nurses must be part of the solution in this endeavor. We must collaborate with physicians and other colleagues in creating processes that assist in narrowing the communication gap for all our pediatric patients and families.

How can nurses ensure that they have the tools, resources, and fundamental knowledge base to provide health literate care to the pediatric patient population? With the largest age group of employed nurses now older than age 50, the nursing profession has the responsibility to ensure this workforce is brought up to date on electronic initiatives aimed at improving health literacy. As a generation not typically having an expertise in electronics, this generation of nurses can learn from the younger generation who are more adept with electronics, including laptops, iPhones, and laptop computers.

Encouraging ongoing education and lifelong learning in the nursing profession is vital so that we can prepare our nurses for the future. Currently, only 13.2% of the nursing workforce is masters or doctoral prepared (American Nurses Association, 2011). Educating nurses in health literacy, including plain language, cultural, and linguistic competency, and teach-back techniques, is another important strategy for reducing patient error and improving child safety. A reported study in a pediatric emergency department looked at using a structured educational approach that included use of teach-back methods, patient and medication specific-plain language, pictogram-based medication instruction sheets, and a standardized dosing sheet in discharge medication teaching. The results demonstrated a reduction in dosing errors as compared to their usual practice (Yin et al., 2008).

The United States health care system is in a state of constant change. One of the driving forces for this change is the call for the provision of increased quality of care and patient safety initiatives that will help prevent medical errors, improve quality, and ultimately enhance patient outcomes. In addition, as a result of these initiatives, associated health care costs will decrease. The caregivers to pediatric patients must be able to calculate dosages, read pharmacy labels, and locate specialists for their children. In order to adequately complete these tasks, a high level of health literacy skills is needed. Private agencies and organizations such as the Agency for Healthcare Research and Quality, The Centers for Disease Control and Prevention, and the AAP, must be the leaders for health literacy research and adoption of evidence-based interventions to advance the field (Kutner et al., 2007).

As the health care industry moves toward a more consumer-based health care system, the caregivers need to begin to take a more proactive role in all health decisions for their children. Parents and caregivers are encouraged to develop a personal health record for their children and for themselves. This is the first step toward educating their family on past medical histories, family histories, and drug allergies—all vital information necessary to have when entering any medical facility for health care. The pediatric nurse is encouraged to take a proactive role in educating his or her patients and parents or caregivers. This is everyone's responsibility as we shape the future for our children, grandchildren, and all future generations. Collectively we can reach the goal of improving the safety, outcomes, and overall quality of life for each pediatric patient we serve (Noblin, Wan, & Fottler, 2011).

The need to have educational and informational materials written in plain language, with consideration of reading levels, and translated to the preferred languages of the population served must be a priority. This will enable families and patients to receive information to prevent illness and promote health. Ensuring these brochures, booklets, and applications are readily available in waiting areas, online, and via smart phone will enhance success. The identification of valid assessment tools for children and caregivers to determine their health literacy skills must be improved. In addition, a special focus is needed on children as they transition into young adulthood. As children with chronic illness and other disease states enter adulthood, we must ensure a seamless heath care transition for the patient and the family.

Children are the future of our nation. If we do not ensure the health literacy for this population, they will suffer the consequences of nonaction. It is everyone's responsibility in the health care industry to work toward health literacy for every child and family. Nurses, who make up the largest population of the health care workforce, must make health literacy education and dissemination a priority as the implications to their scope of practice and patient outcome measures are linked. Nurses are leaders. As you read this book you may be a student starting your career, a staff nurse, an assistant nurse manger, a nurse manager, a chief nursing officer, or a nurse in the midst of planning for retirement. Wherever you are in your career, health literacy and ensuring its evolution will only enhance your career and the outcomes attainable. There is still much to be done. Additional research is needed to enhance our understanding of health literacy and the implications with child and family health outcomes and costs of care (Wilson, Brown, & Stephens-Ferris, 2006). By focusing on health literacy issues we can improve the accessibility, quality, and safety of health care; reduce costs; and improve the health and quality of life for millions of children and adults in the United States (U.S. Department of Health and Human Services, National Action Plan, 2010).

References

Abrams, M. A., Klass, P., & Dreyer, B. P. (2009). Health literacy and children: Introduction. *Pediatrics, 124,* S262–S264.

Abrams, M. A., Klass, P., & Dreyer, B. P. (2009). Health literacy and children: Recommendations for action. *Pediatrics, 124,* S327–S331.

American Nurses Association. (2011). *American Nurses Association fact sheet.* Retrieved from www.NursingWorld.org

Bloom, B., Cohen, R. A., & Freeman, G. (2012). Summary health statistics for U.S. children: National Health Interview Survey, 2011. National Center for Health Statistics. *Vital Health Statistics, 10*(254).

Boice, M. (1998). Chronic illness in adolescence. *Adolescence, 33,* 927–934.

Borzekowski, D. (2009). Considering children and health literacy: A theoretical approach. *Pediatrics, 124,* 282–288.

Davis, T. C., Wolf, M. S., Arnold, C. L., Byrd, R. S., Long, S. W., Springer, T., . . . Bocchini, J. A. (2006). Development and validation of the Rapid Estimate of Adolescent Literacy in Medicine (REALM-Teen): A tool to screen adolescents for below-grade reading in health care settings. *Pediatrics, 118,* e1707–e1714.

Doak, C., Doak, L., & Root, J. (1996). *Teaching patients with low literacy skills* (2nd ed.). Philadelphia, PA: J. B. Lippincott.

Flowers, L. (2006). Teach-back improves informed consent. *OR Manager, 22*(3), 25–26.

Fredrickson, D. D., Washington, R. L., Pham, N., Jackson, T., Wiltshire, J., & Jecha, L. D. (1995). Reading grade levels and health behaviors of parents at child clinics. *Kansas Medicine, 96*(3), 127–129.

Kutner, M., Greenberg, E., Jin, Y., Boyle, B., Hsu, Y., & Dunleavy, E. (2007). *Literacy in everyday life: Results from the 2003 National Assessment of Adult Literacy* (NCES 2007-480), U.S. Department of Education. Washington, DC: National Center for Education Statistics.

Kutner, M., Greenberg, E., Jin, Y., & Paulsen, C. (2006). *The health literacy of America's adults: Results from the 2003 National Assessment of Adult Literacy* (NCES Publication No. 2006-483). U.S. Department of Education. Washington, DC: National Center for Education Statistics.

Lokker, N., Sanders, L., Perrin, E. M., Kumar, D., Finkle, J., Franco, V., . . . Rothman, R. L. (2009). Parental misinterpretations of over the counter pediatric cough and cold medication labels. *Pediatrics, 123*(6), 1464–1471.

Manganello, J. A. (2007). Health literacy and adolescents: A framework and agenda for future research. *Health Education Research, 23*(5), 840–847. Retrieved from http://her.oxfordjournals.gov

Monsen, R. B. (2007). Child health literacy. *Journal of Pediatric Nursing, 22*(1), 69–70.

Mosby's Medical Dictionary (8th ed.). (2009). St. Louis, MO: Elsevier.

National Center for Education Statistics. (2005). *The condition of education 2006* (NCES Publication No. 2005-014). Washington, DC: U.S. Department of Education.

Nielsen-Bohlman, L., Panzar, A., & Kindig, D. A. (2004). *Health literacy: A prescription to end confusion.* Washington, DC: The National Academies Press.

Noblin, A. M., Wan, T. T. H., & Fottler, M. (2011). The impact of health literacy on a patient's decision to adopt a personal health record. *Perspectives in health information management.* Retrieved from Perspectives.ahima.org

Nutbeam, D. (2000). Health literacy as a public health goal: A challenge for contemporary health education and communication strategies in the 21st century. *Health Promotion International, 15*, 259–268.

Raver, R, Hancock, M., & Ingersoll, G. (2004). Online forum messages posted by adolescents with type 1 diabetes. *Diabetes Educator, 30*, 827–834.

Roter, D. (2000). The medical visit context of treatment decision-making and the therapeutic relationship. *Health Expectations, 3*(1), 17–25.

Rothman, R. L., Housman, R., Weiss, H., Davis, D., Gregory, R., Gebretsadik, T., . . . Elasy, T. A. (2006). Patient understanding of food labels: The role of literacy and numeracy. *American Journal of Preventive Medicine, 31*(5), 391–398.

Rothman, R. L., Yin, H. S., Mulvaney, S., Co, J. P. T., Homer, C., & Lannon, C. (2009). Health literacy and quality: Focus on chronic illness care and patient safety. *Pediatrics, 124*, S315.

Sanders, L. M., Federico, S., Klass, P., Abrams, M. A., & Dreyer, B. (2009). Literacy and child health: A systematic review. *Archives of Pediatrics and Adolescent Medicine, 162*(4), 131–138.

Sanders, L. M., Shaw, J. S., Guez, G., Baur, C., & Rudd, R. (2009). Health literacy and child health promotion: Implications for research, clinical care, and public policy. *Pediatrics, 124*, 306–314.

Sanders, L. M., Thompson, V. T., & Wilkinson, J. D. (2007). Caregiver health literacy and the use of child health services. *Pediatrics, 119*(1), 86–92.

Turner, T., Cull, W. L., Bayldon, B., Klass, P., Sanders, L. M., Frintner, M. P., . . . Dreyer, B. (2009). Pediatricians and health literacy: Descriptive results from a national survey. *Pediatrics, 124,* 299–305.

U.S. Census. (2010). *Age and sex composition: 2010.* Retrieved from http://www .census.gov/prod/cen2010/briefs/c2010br-03.pdf

U.S. Department of Health and Human Services, Office of Disease Prevention and Health Promotion. (2010). *National action plan to improve health literacy.* Washington, DC: Author.

Vilella, A., Bavas, J. M., Diaz, M. T., Guinovart, C., Diez, C., Simo, D., & Cerezo, J. (2004). The role of mobile phones in improving vaccination rates in travelers. *Preventive Medicine, 28*(4), 503–509.

Wilson, F. L., Brown, D. L., & Stephens-Ferris, M. (2006). Can easy to read immunization information increase knowledge in urban low-income mothers? *Journal of Pediatric Nursing, 21,* 4–12.

Wittich, A. R., Mangan, J., Grad, R., Wand, W., & Gerald, L. B. (2007). Pediatric asthma: Caregiver health literacy and the clinician's perception. *Journal of Asthma, 44*(1), 51–55.

Wolff, K., Cavanaugh, K., Malone, R., Hawk, V., Gregory, B. P., Davis, D., . . . Rothman, R. L. (2009). The Diabetes Literacy and Numeracy Education Toolkit: Materials to facilitate diabetes education and management in patients with low literacy and numeracy skills. *Diabetes Educator, 35*(2), 233–236, 238–241, 244–245.

Yin, H. S., Dreyer, B. P., van Schaick, L., Foltin, G. L., Dinglas, C., & Mendelsohn, A. L. (2008). Randomized controlled trial of a pictogram-based intervention to reduce liquid medication dosing error and improve adherence among caregivers of young children. *Archives of Pediatric and Adolescent Medicine, 162*(9), 814–822.

Yin, H. S., Johnson, M., Mendelsohn, A. L., Abrams, M. A., Sanders, L. M., & Dreyer, B. P. (2009). The health literacy of parents in the United States: A nationally representative study. *Pediatrics, 124*(Suppl. 3), S289–S298.

13

Mental Health Disorders

Fallon Edwards

Case Scenario

John is a 34-year-old married male. He is a very high-powered executive in one of the country's top health systems with a very demanding schedule. John is also a doctoral candidate at an Ivy League school, working toward his PhD in health economics with a focus in urban communities. He has very high standards for himself and can be very self-critical when he fails to meet them. This is a result of growing up in a household where his parents held very high standards for him, but not his three sisters. They were very reprimanding when he did not meet their standards. He graduated with top honors in both college and graduate school. Unfortunately, he is failing to meet his expected high standards in his current doctoral program, and is continuously struggling with overwhelming feelings of embarrassment and insignificance due to his inability to perform as well as he has most of his life.

Over the past few weeks, John has felt unusually lethargic and his work performance has declined. His coworkers have noticed that he is not as social and closes his office door more often, which is very unlike him. His colleagues noticed his changed behavior when he started calling out sick frequently and not responding to e-mails when he's out of the office, which is the complete

241

opposite of his typical behavior. On the days that he stays home, he's usually on his couch or in the bed all day sleeping or watching television.

John's wife has noticed that he has changed at home also. He no longer plays with his two young kids for any more than 5 minutes when he gets home from work. Over the past few weeks, he has shown little interest in sex and does not get much sleep. His constant position switching between sitting up and lying in the bed often awakens his wife. When she looks at him, he is always staring at the ceiling. Quite a few times, the sound of him sobbing in their master bathroom with the door closed has awakened her too. She tried several times to get him to speak to her about what's bothering him and each time he says, "I'm fine," rather quickly and leaves the room that they are in.

John is very unhappy with his life, but he has never considered committing suicide. He often wishes he were dead. John gets very aggravated with himself because he knows he should be happy, but allows his disappointment in himself for not excelling in his doctoral program to overwhelm him.

About Mental Health Disorders

As in the story of John, most mental disorders are greatly associated with suicidal behavior, but it is depression that is considered the most relevant contributing disorder. Psychological autopsy studies have shown that approximately 60% of people who commit suicide had a significant depressive disorder (Chamberlain, Goldney, Taylor, & Eckert, 2012, p. 525). Prevalence estimates suggest that in the United States, depression affects 6.6% of adults each year (Wang & Lai, 2008, p. 191) and approximately 50% of adults over a lifetime (Swami, Papanicolaou, & Furnham, 2011, p. 662). Recent studies have highlighted the significance of major depression as a contributing factor to both attempted suicide and thoughts of committing suicide (Chamberlain et al., 2012, p. 525). "By 2030, depression is projected to be the number one cause of disability, ahead of cardiovascular disease, traffic accidents, chronic pulmonary disease, and HIV/AIDS" (Kazdin & Rabbitt, 2013, p. 171).

Anxiety disorders are a risk factor for substance use (Coles & Coleman, 2010, p. 63). Independently and collectively, they are major health problems in the United States. Anxiety disorders will affect approximately 18% of adults annually and 28% of adults during their lifetimes. They are the most expensive mental health disorder, costing the United States over $40 billion annually. Anxiety disorders also account for approximately 31% of all mental health costs.

Additionally, they can begin at early ages and their chronic nature increases their negative impact (Coles & Coleman, 2010, p. 63). Substance abuse disorders impact over 20 million Americans and costs approximately $500 billion annually in the United States (Kazdin & Rabbitt, 2013, p. 171). Mental health disorders not only have a significant impact on the individuals who are diagnosed with them, but when coupled with other psychiatric disorders, they cause a major financial burden on the economy.

Although this information focused on only a few mental health disorders, as a whole they are rather common among the general public. In the United States, approximately 25% of the population, which is about 79 million people, in any given year meets the criteria for having a mental health disorder. Approximately 30% of the world's population is estimated to have at least one mental health disorder in a 12-month period (Kazdin & Rabbitt, 2013, p. 171). The percentage of the privately insured population who use a psychiatric drug grew from 13.7% in 1998 to 20% in 2009 (Mark, Levit, Vandivort-Warren, Buck, & Coffey, 2011, p. 287). In 2005, the United States spent approximately $113 billion on mental health treatment (Mark et al., 2011, p. 285). The high incidence of mental health disorders worldwide is an important public health concern due to its significant emotional, physical, and economic impact on individuals and families, and the socioeconomic burden on national economies (Swami et al., 2011, pp. 662–663).

Significance of Mental Health Disorders to Health Literacy

Health literacy (see Chapter 1, "Health Literacy: History, Definitions, and Models") was applied to the realm of mental health disorders in which the term mental health literacy was developed by Jorm in 1997, and defined as the "knowledge and beliefs about mental disorders which aid their recognition, management or prevention." Similar to health literacy, mental health literacy has the following components: "(1) recognition of specific disorders or different types of psychological distress; (2) knowledge and beliefs about risk factors and causes; (3) knowledge and beliefs about professional help available; (4) attitudes which facilitate recognition and appropriate help-seeking; and (5) knowledge of how to seek mental health information" (Jorm, 2000, p. 396).

Mental health literacy is typically assessed by using Jorm's questionnaire. The questionnaire consists of a vignette with either a male (John) or female (Mary) character who displays classical features of depression. The vignette is told using the same gender character as the gender of the questionnaire's respondent. Respondents were asked in an open-ended format what they thought was wrong with the person, and what type of help the person could seek. They were able to give as many answers as they liked. Respondents were asked about the helpfulness of specific interventions. They were also asked about contact with individuals who had similar symptoms displayed in the vignette, and whether they ever had similar symptoms or ever sought treatment for them. Research findings from the assessments using this vignette have found that mental health literacy is an important determinant of help-seeking behavior (Chamberlain et al., 2012, p. 528). If individuals with mental health disorders do not know the signs and symptoms of their own mental health disorders, how will they know when to seek treatment? Results from several studies have shown that people with low health literacy are three times more likely to have depression, although low health literacy was not an independent risk factor for depression (Lincoln et al., 2006, p. 821). The millions of individuals who experience both a mental health disorder (depression will be used as an example due to its previously discussed significance) and low health literacy also face a double challenge, as they have to manage two demanding health characteristics that have the same barriers to treatment and implications. The barriers to treatment for people with depression are that persons with depression do not recognize that they are in need of treatment, stigma, refusal to believe that treatments are effective, inability to afford medical attention, and structural barriers (i.e., inconvenience, unable to make an appointment) (Mojtabai et al., 2011, pp. 1751–1752). The barriers to treatment for people with low health literacy are: shame and stigma, increased health care costs, minimum knowledge about illnesses and treatments, and less access to care (see Chapter 2, "Low Health Literacy and Implications"). The barriers to treatment for both groups are compared in Table 13.1.

Shame and Stigma

Shame and stigma both relate to the feelings individuals have about themselves or others. Individuals with mental health disorders typically have limited reading ability, which can result in high levels of shame and is likely to result in the display of depressive symptoms (Lincoln et al., 2011, p. 822). When individuals experience shame, they typically do not want to discuss this feeling with others. Holding in these feelings does not allow individuals to overcome their shame because they typically do not seek help—even those close to these individuals cannot help since they are not aware of these feelings. These individuals live in

Table 13.1 Comparison of Barriers to Treatment for Mental Health and Illness and Health Literacy

Mental Health and Illness	Health Literacy
• Not recognizing that in their current state they are in need of treatment	• Minimum knowledge about illnesses and treatments
• Stigma	• Shame and stigma
• Refusing to believe that treatments are effective	• Minimum knowledge about illnesses and treatments
• Inability to afford medical attention	• Increased health care costs
• Structural barriers (i.e., inconvenience, unable to make an appointment)	• Less access to care

fear that their limited reading ability will be exposed if they have to interact with medical professionals, resulting in feelings of shame.

The form of stigma typically related to individuals with mental health disorder is personal stigma, which is "an individual's personal attitudes towards the person with mental illness" (Wang & Lai, 2008, p. 192). Unlike shame, stigmatizing attitudes are well known by both those who are performing the act of stigmatizing and those with mental health disorders. Large-scale educational campaigns developed across the United States to address and minimize stigma about people with mental health disorders were unsuccessful. Providing education on topics that people have minimum knowledge about always seem to be the best route in assisting them to making more rational decisions. However, stigmatizing attitudes toward people with mental health disorders differ so much from person to person, that it has been difficult for educational campaigns to focus on a number of stigmatizing attitudes and successfully educate a significant portion of the target audience (Wang & Lai, 2008, p. 192). For the most part, stigma is what prevents individuals with mental health disorders from possibly receiving medical treatment.

Increased Health Care Costs

The billions of dollars a year mental health disorders cost the United States, combined with the billions of dollars a year low health literacy costs the

United States (see Chapter 1, "Health Literacy: History, Definitions, and Models"), result in a major financial concern not only for the economy and the health care system, but also for individuals. These large dollar figures are mainly a representation of the large and continuously growing number of people with mental health disorders who have an ever-growing need for medical assistance. They will have to seek more medical attention and possibly have to take more medicines.

In relation to health literacy, patient education resources for the different types of mental health disorders should be created, providers need to be educated on how to speak in plain language when discussing mental health disorders terminology, and understandable signage with correct lay terminology should be created for facilities that offer services for mental health disorders. Although each of these initiatives is crucial to meeting the needs of those with mental health disorders, they will lead to an increase in spending.

There are millions of uninsured people who have a mental health disorder. Health care services are very costly, and not having health insurance typically leads to poor health outcomes as a result of not being able to afford medical services. The 2008 National Survey on Drug Use and Health states that 4.9 million uninsured people had serious psychological distress in the past year (Mark et al., 2011, p. 290). People with mental health disorders who had limits on their psychiatric and substance abuse health insurance benefits should be able to gain better access to services as a result of the Paul Wellstone and Pete Domenici Mental Health Parity and Addiction Equity Act of 2008. Additionally, Medicaid is the largest payer of mental illness treatments (Mark et al., 2011, p. 288). The Patient Protection and Affordable Care Act of 2010 will benefit those with mental health disorders due to the Medicaid expansions (Mark et al., 2011, p. 290). Since mental health disorders occur mostly in people with limited resources, and because their health state often leads to diminished income, employment opportunities, and insurance coverage, they usually have the least access to treatments and services. They are also more likely to have low health literacy since they have not had much experience with seeking medical attention and navigating the health care system.

Poor Health Outcomes

Individuals with low health literacy are more likely to be in poor health (see Chapter 2, "Low Health Literacy and Implications"). In Lincoln et al.'s (2006) study, which looked at the relationship between health literacy and mental health outcomes, "low health literacy was found to be associated with higher levels of depressive symptoms" (p. 820). In addition, the participants with low health literacy were three times more likely to have depression (Lincoln et al., 2006, p. 821). This in itself explains how enhancing the health literacy of persons with mental health disorders will make a grand impact in the mental health realm. The other barriers to treatment discussed in this section also equally contribute to the poor health outcomes of people with mental health disorders.

Minimum Knowledge About Illnesses and Treatments

The major burden of mental health disorders is the significant proportion of adults who do not receive any treatment because they do not recognize mental health disorders and do not understand the meanings of psychiatric terms. In Mojtabai et al.'s (2011) study, the most common barrier to treatment across all levels of severity of any mental health disorder was not feeling there was a need for treatment (p. 1757). The majority of those who recognized a need for treatment but who did not seek treatment, believed that their state of health was not severe or that it would get better on its own. When individuals are not aware of all of the facts about their health state, signs, symptoms, and how to seek treatment, it's hard for them to know when and how to seek medical attention.

Less Use of Preventive Services

An important factor for people with mental health disorders to receive the medical attention they need is to increase access to preventive services. Approximately 70% of people with mental health disorders who are in need of treatment do not receive it (Kazdin & Rabbitt, 2013, p. 171). If there is such a large percentage of people not receiving treatments, then there is likely a similar percentage of people not using preventive services, since the use of preventive services would lessen the need for eventually needing treatment. This is not only due to the factors previously discussed such as shame, stigma, unaffordability of medical services, and lack of knowledge, but also due to the delivery method of health care services. The delivery method available may not be accessible. Inaccessible services could be location. For example, Mike has schizophrenia, his closest family members live at least 2 hours away from him, and he does not drive. Since he works Monday through Friday, he schedules his medical appointments on the weekends. There is a bus stop three blocks away from his house that can take him to a medical facility where he can receive his treatments. However, on the weekends, the bus only runs every hour. Most times

Mike is unable to schedule his appointments during times that will lessen his travel or wait time. There were times when he was finished with his appointments a few minutes after the bus left and he would have to wait almost an hour for the next bus. After 6 weeks of treatments, Mike stopped going. If the health care facility were in walking distance it would be more accessible, but the travel and wait times make his medical treatments inconvenient.

In addition, the delivery method available may not be the most effective. The way medical information is communicated and who provides the medical services can make the delivery method of preventive services ineffective for people with mental health disorders. Some examples of ineffective delivery methods include patients who actually have the transportation means and health insurance coverage to go to doctor visits or treatment programs, but do not understand the information that is being communicated to them. Another example is having nationally recognized and scientifically proven effective online self-help programs available free to everyone who experiences the same mental illness, but limited reading ability does not make it feasible to complete a 12-hour online program containing just text—no pictures and no sound. Another example, which is the current situation, is having highly trained mental health professionals but not enough of them are in locations accessible to those in need, and they are not culturally representative of the populations they serve.

Implications of Low Health Literacy to Mental Health Disorders

In the realm of mental health disorders, nursing practice can greatly benefit from applying the tenets of health literacy, or mental health literacy, in the effort to enhance the health care experience for themselves, their patients, and society. As nurses increase their knowledge of mental health disorders, it will enhance their skill set in preventing, diagnosing, and seeking appropriate treatment options for their patients with these disorders, and in patient safety. This will also result in an increase in access to medical treatments when the delivery method of task shifting is used. This is when more nurses are placed on the front line of providing medical care to specific populations, such as people with mental health disorders.

Recognition of Specific Disorders or Different Types of Psychological Distress

Creating a shame-free environment or using open-ended questions (see Chapter 4, "The Health Literacy Environment: Enhancing Access and Wayfinding)" to find out more about why a patient is seeking medical care, can assist in possibly determining if the patient has a mental health disorder. Even if patients identify that they have a mental health disorder, they may not know which one they have as studies have shown that people misunderstand psychological terms such as "schizophrenia," "mania," and "psychopathy" (Swami et al., 2011, p. 663). Using plain language and teach-back will enhance patient–provider communication, and ensure that accurate information is being transmitted to the patient. Nurses, as well as other health care professionals, are accustomed to speaking in medical terminology. However, the use of plain language, in which simple and basic words and concepts are used, will make the patient feel comfortable and result in an open dialogue where the nurse can use teach-back to confirm understanding (see Chapter 6, "Effective Communication and Plain Language").

Nurses and their patients with mental health disorders can build a strong communication relationship when the foundation includes accurate information about the state of the patient's health. Since most people are unaware of the symptoms of mental health disorders, it is unlikely that patients will believe that they have a psychological problem, and therefore not explain their symptoms in that manner. As a result, this often leads to nurses not making an inference toward mental health since the information was not communicated in that manner. Nurses' awareness of how people perceive the cause of mental health disorders, patients' use of incorrect psychiatric labels and terminology, and not being aware of symptoms will better prepare nurses in communicating, diagnosing, and developing treatment plans for their patients with mental health disorders.

Knowledge and Beliefs About Risk Factors and Causes

Cultural influences play a major role in how people believe mental health disorders are caused. In the Western countries, people feel that depression and schizophrenia are caused by the social environment, mainly recent stressors. In non-Western countries, people believe that mental illnesses are caused by supernatural phenomena (i.e., witchcraft) and possession by evil spirits. Across many different countries, people have very negative beliefs about medicine for various mental illnesses. This is in contrast to the results from randomized controlled trials and the perspectives of mental health professionals that various types of medicines are effective (Jorm, 2000, p. 397).

If nurses are not knowledgeable in cultural beliefs regarding causation and symptoms of mental health disorders, it is likely that their communication may not be effective as they may have different beliefs about the causation of mental health disorders. The way patients explain their health history and symptoms to their nurses may not be how their nurses believe mental health disorders are caused or that their patients even have a mental health disorder.

Knowledge and Beliefs About Available Professional Help

Society's opinions about the efficacy of psychiatric and psychological treatments also differ from those of health practitioners. Patients and society, which include the family members and friends of patients, both prefer self-help and alternative treatment options over conventional methods (Jorm, 2000; Swami et al., 2011). The most popular self-help option is looking to family members and friends for support. This is important for nurses to know as they can tailor their education not only to their patients, but also to their patients' family members and friends. Health literacy plays a major role in this respect as society is not knowledgeable about the various aspects pertaining to mental health disorders. Studies have confirmed that societies as a whole are not knowledgeable about how to deal with people with mental health disorders because they are afraid of making mistakes.

Since it's well known that people with mental health disorders look to their family members and friends for help and support, but the family members and friends are not comfortable dealing with their state of health, then this is a process that needs to be addressed. For all parties to receive any type of benefit out of this "support" structure, patients with mental health disorders must seek help and support from nurses and other health practitioners, as they are likely to be more knowledge about mental health disorders and identify symptoms at an earlier stage. In addition, when nurses include family members and friends into their patients' treatment plans it can lead to higher treatment completion rates, as patients with mental health disorders perceive their families' and friends' help to be very important and seek help from them first. In turn, nurses will find it easier to customize their education style to determine what type of treatment options their patients prefer and learn to incorporate their preferences into developing an appropriate treatment plan, as a patient with a mental health disorder treatment preference may be different than a patient with a different type of health condition. Clearly explaining the treatment plan to patients so they are able to understand the information will allow patients to become more comfortable and open to attempting other help-seeking and treatment options, such as conventional methods.

Attitudes That Facilitate Recognition and Appropriate Help-Seeking

An important aspect to increase the number of people with mental health disorders who receive medical attention is to understand why this population either does not seek or complete their treatment. Only approximately 25% of people with anxiety disorders and approximately 40% of people with mood disorders seek treatment within the first year after onset. Almost all of the anxiety disorders have an average treatment delay that exceeds 10 years (Coles & Coleman, 2010, p. 64). Of the small portion of people with mental health disorders who receive treatment, many of them drop out before completing their treatment. Unfortunately, the majority of those who drop out are individuals with severe cases of mental illness.

The high occurrence of people judging their need for treatment incorrectly is one factor why patients and the public need to be accurately educated on the signs of severe mental health disorders and the appropriate treatment options. Nurses caring for patients with mental health disorders will benefit greatly while providing medical attention when they are well educated on the advanced or severe signs and symptoms, due to patients' delay in treatment seeking. Since it's well known that society as a whole is unfamiliar with the different types and signs and symptoms of mental illnesses, this affects help-seeking behavior to the point where patients do not seek medical attention until their mental illness is at an advanced stage, when the signs and symptoms are severe. This will require that nurses are educated beyond basic knowledge, and know how to educate their patients so they are able to understand the severity of their health state and the advanced treatment options for their particular mental illness.

Patient Safety

Patient safety is a major component in the realm of mental health disorders in situations where there is a near miss, or a delay or error in care, due to lack of hand-off communication from provider to provider. Near misses are learning opportunities used with no-harm events to act as guides for health system improvements. In health care, near misses occur approximately 3 to 300 times more often than adverse events, which are linked to a negative outcome or harm to the patient. As part of their accreditation process, health care organizations are required to show that they made improvements as a result of lessons learned from reported near-misses (Jeffs, Macrae, Maione, & Macmillan, 2012, p. 431).

Medication errors are a prime example of near misses in mental health disorders. Substance abuse disorders are highly prevalent among patients with mental health disorders due to the many medications these patients take at any given time (Mark et al., 2011, p. 284). The high number of medications makes it common for important information to be missed during hand-off communication. An example is a patient with a mental health disorder starting to display a new and potentially harmful behavior after being on a particular pill for 3 days. The patient's nurse noticed the behavior change and alerted the patient's psychiatrist. Because the patient was taking six different medications, it was not apparent to the nurse that the medication could have been the cause of this new behavior. After the nurse and psychiatrist reviewed the patient's medical record together, they noticed the time when the patient began this new medication correlated with the onset of the patient's new behavior. The new medication was somehow not mentioned during hand-off communication, but the psychiatrist took the patient off of that particular pill, and gave him a new pill that does not have that side effect. Fortunately, the nurse and psychiatrist were able to observe this behavior and intercede before the patient could do any harm. The omission of or delay in providing information about the new medication could have resulted in a harmful outcome, but that was avoided.

In an effort to prepare future nurses to detect safety risks among people with mental health disorders, studies have shown that particular competencies should be used in the education curriculum. These study results have led to the development of two sets of patient safety competencies. These two competencies can be built upon to show relevance to this population and are called the Canadian Patient Safety Institute Safety Competencies and the Robert Wood Johnson Foundation Quality and Safety Education for Nurse (QSEN) Competencies. (Jeffs et al., 2012, p. 436)

Task Shifting

There is a lack of mental health professionals to reach the unserved. In the United States, mental health professionals are typically found in highly dense, affluent urban areas and in cities where major universities are located. Ironically, studies have shown that having a high income is associated with positive attitudes toward mental health disorders treatments (Mojtabai et al., 2011, p. 1758). The majority of people with mental health disorders live in rural areas and small towns, and obviously not in close proximity to where most mental health professionals are located. In addition, the majority of mental health professionals do not provide care for clinical problems and populations where there is a great need, such as adolescents and children, and an expanding need, such as the elderly. Most importantly, younger people tend to have more of a negative perspective toward mental health treatment seeking. Additionally, people age 65 and above are typically covered by Medicare and are retired. Therefore, they are more likely not to have financial and time barriers, but still tend to lack a perceived need for treatment (Mojtabai et al., 2011, p. 1758). Overall, there are not enough mental health professionals trained to provide services to these populations. Lastly, there is only a small portion of mental health professionals, including nurses, who reflect the cultures and ethnicities of the populations in need of care (Kazdin & Rabbitt, 2013, p. 172). Those who reflect the cultures and ethnicities typically are not trained in the communities where these populations are located.

The limited reach of mental health professionals and limited access for people with mental health disorders in the one-to-one, in-person process of delivering services will clearly not have much of an impact even if the workforce is increased. This is evident in the approximately 700,000 mental health professionals in relation to the approximately 79 million people in the United States who meet the criteria for having a mental health disorder in any given year (Kazdin & Rabbitt, 2013, p. 171). This has resulted in the United States placing more focus on task shifting with nurses in the area of mental health.

Task shifting is a way of redistributing the delivery of services to a broad range of people with less training and fewer qualifications than a traditional health care worker to strengthen and expand the health care workforce. In the case of mental health disorders, task shifting can be used to train nurses who are not knowledgeable and do not work with the mental health population. This practice is not new and is currently occurring in countries such as the United States, Australia, and England where nurses, nurse assistants, and pharmacologists provide services that were once reserved for doctors. In the United States, mental health professionals with advanced training (masters or doctoral level) in one-to-one, in-person sessions administer many treatment options for mental health disorders (Kazdin & Rabbitt, 2013, pp. 171–172). This method of delivering treatment options is dominant in providing evidence-based interventions, and is always in high demand. However, this method of delivering treatment does not reach many underserved people with mental health disorders, but with task shifting, access to this treatment method will increase. With proper training given to nurses, task shifting can greatly reduce or eliminate barriers to treatment for people with mental health disorders and low health literacy skills.

Task shifting works well in the mental health realm because of its ability to be scaled up to provide services to the unserved, and its adaptability to diverse countries, communities, and cultures. This was shown in the results of a randomized control trial of treatment of anxiety and depression in India using tasking shifting. The results showed that lay counselors could be successfully trained to manage treatment options with reliability. It also showed that the prevalence of mental health disorders in a large sample was reduced through the interventions that were administered (Kazdin & Rabbitt, 2013, p. 174). This confirms that, certainly in developing countries, task shifting is feasible, is beyond the planning stages and ready for widespread implementation to nurses in the mental health realm.

In addition to task shifting, care for mental health disorders has shifted from psychiatric hospitals to general hospital psychiatric units over the past 20 years. By 2005, a larger amount of spending for mental health disorders was for treatment in general hospitals. In addition, most spending for treatments go to providers that are specially trained to treat mental health disorders (Mark et al., 2011, p. 288). Nursing curricula and ongoing nursing education should prepare all nurses with the knowledge on how to care for patients with mental health disorders as care and treatment is evolving into various settings and the amount of patients are rapidly growing, as seen from the projection that depression will become the number one cause of disability by 2030 (Kazdin & Rabbitt, 2013, p. 171). In general, 25% of Americans, or 79 million people, will have a mental health disorder each year.

As a result, millions of people with mental health disorders will enter the health care system each year and will likely have minimal knowledge about their disorder and low health literacy skills; nurses can be prepared for this with the proper training.

Summary

The high lifetime prevalence of mental health disorders essentially means that almost everyone will either have a mental health disorder or know someone who does. Jorm's creation of the term mental health literacy, which branches off of health literacy, drew attention to society's lack of knowledge of mental health disorders and all health care professionals, including nurses, lack of understanding of society's beliefs and viewpoints toward mental health disorders. Low mental health literacy affects everyone from the layperson to the health care professional. Addressing the barriers in mental health disorders and in low health literacy, will provide an increase in knowledge and seeking and accessing treatment options.

Research has shown that low health literacy was associated with higher levels of depressive symptoms (Lincoln et al., 2006, p. 820). If people with mental illnesses seek medical treatments, it is usually done after long delays. Most people do not seek medical treatment because they are unable to recognize and identify the symptoms of mental illnesses (Coles & Coleman, 2010, p. 64). Increasing health literacy skills in people who are depressed and suicidal should make them more aware of the signs and symptoms of mental health disorders and, in turn, lead to more people seeking treatment. As a result, the incidence of suicide caused by depression, and the prevalence of all other mental illnesses, should decrease. Additionally, if patients have more accurate knowledge about medicines for their mental health disorder, they may be more likely to comply with their treatment regimen. This will also assist in providing them with a more positive outlook on the efficacy of medicine options.

Another reason why they may not seek medical treatment is that their preferred form of intervention is self-help, where they typically seek information from family members and friends. Since society is also not very knowledgeable about mental health disorders and the treatment options, this form of intervention is not very beneficial in producing favorable results. Increasing potential patients' and society's knowledge about mental health disorders will increase the likelihood that they will seek medical treatments, and at an early stage.

Increased knowledge of mental health disorders also enhances patient–provider communication. The patient's use of correct psychiatric terminology and knowing the signs and symptoms along with nurses knowing society's perspectives and cultural beliefs toward mental health disorders, will allow both the patient and nurse to communicate with a clear understanding of each other. The nurse's concern with how patients are motivated to learn will assist patients in feeling comfortable to make their own health care decisions based upon their interests. The communication will be most effective if both the patient and nurse combine their perspectives to come to mutually agreeable decisions that are also effective in producing enhanced outcomes.

A review of the data on why people with mental health disorders either don't seek treatment, begin treatment but don't complete it, or wait until they show severe signs and symptoms of their illness shows that it is not always a result of the available treatment options. The delivery of treatment options is an important issue in the accessibility, affordability, and the ability to scale up services to reach people in need. Focusing efforts on expanding task shifting will result in more health care professionals becoming available to provide mental health services, an increase in access to care for patients, and lessen the burden of mental illness worldwide. An increase in access to treatment options will lead to a growth in treatment spending due to more people with mental health disorders seeking treatment options. However, this cost is minimal in comparison to the cost of hospitalizations, hospital readmissions, and high usage of the emergency department.

Incorporating patient safety competencies into nursing education will improve patient safety outcomes in the mental health and illness population. Knowing how to detect safety risks and providing the safest possible care will have a huge impact on how society perceives mental illness treatment options and their comfort level with health care professionals who provide mental health services. Quality of care is a factor patients use in determining if they want to seek help and if they feel comfortable interacting with health care professionals.

The mental health population is very complex and has many variables to consider when educating patients on prevention, signs and symptoms, and treatment options. The same holds true when society and health care professionals are learning about the mental health population. Using the tenets of health literacy when addressing the five components of mental health literacy, discussed earlier in this chapter, works favorably to enhance the medical care and outcomes for this population. Legislation and health policy changes will improve affordability and access to mental health services and treatment options such as the Paul Wellstone and Pete Domenici Mental Health Parity and Addiction Equity Act of 2008 and the Affordable Care Act of 2010. Overall, the use of a patient-centered collaborative approach will make both patients with mental health disorders and nurses feel like a team, working together to produce the most optimal health outcomes.

References

Chamberlain, P. N., Goldney, R. D., Taylor, A. W., & Eckert, K. A. (2012). Have mental health education programs influenced the mental health literacy of those with major depression and suicidal ideation? A comparison between 1998 and 2008 in South Australia. *The Official Journal of the American Association of Suicidology, 42*(5), 525–540. doi:10.1111/j.1943-278X.2012.00109.x

Coles, M. E., & Coleman, S. L. (2010). Barriers to treatment seeking for anxiety disorders: Initial data on the role of mental health literacy. *Depression and Anxiety, 27,* 63–71. doi:10.1002/da.20620

Jeffs, L., Macrae, C., Maione, M., & Macmillan, K. M. (2012). What near misses tell us about risk and safety in mental health care. *Journal of Psychiatric and Mental Health Nursing, 19,* 430–437. doi:10.1111/j.1365-2850.2011.01812.x

Jorm, A. F. (2000). Mental health literacy: Public knowledge and beliefs about mental disorders. *The British Journal of Psychiatry, 177*(5), 396–401. doi:10.1192/bjp.177.5.396

Kazdin, A. E., & Rabbitt, S. M. (2013). Novel models for delivering mental health services and reducing the burdens of mental illness. *Clinical Psychological Science, 1*(2), 170–191. doi:10.1177/2167702612463566

Lincoln, A., Paasche-Orlow, M. K., Cheng, D. M., Lloyd-Travaglini, C., Caruso, C., Saitz, R., & Samet, J. H. (2006). Impact of health literacy on depressive symptoms and mental health-related quality of life among adults with addiction. *Journal of General Internal Medicine, 21,* 818–822. doi:10.111/j.1525-1497.2006.00533.x

Mark, T. L., Levit, K. R., Vandivort-Warren, R., Buck, J. A., & Coffey, R. M. (2011). Changes in US spending on mental health and substance abuse treatment, 1986–2005, and implications for policy. *Health Affairs, 30*(2), 284–292. doi:10.1377/hlthaff.2010.0765

Mojtabai, R., Olfson, M., Sampson, N. A., Jin, R., Druss, B., Wang, P. S., . . . Kessler, R. C. (2011). Barriers to mental health treatment: Results from the National Comorbidity Survey Replication. *Psychological Medicine, 41,* 1751–1761. doi:10.1017/S0033291710002291

Swami, V., Papanicolaou, A., & Furnham, A. (2011). Examining mental health literacy and its correlates using the overclaiming technique. *British Journal of Psychology, 102,* 662–675. doi:10.1111/j.2044-8295.2011.02036.x

Wang, J., & Lai, D. (2008). The relationship between mental health literacy, personal contacts and personal stigma against depression. *Journal of Affective Disorders, 110,* 191–196. doi:10.1016/j.jad.2008.01.005

14

Older Adults

Elizabeth C. McCulloch

Case Scenario

Mr. M is a 74-year-old retired college professor. He has just returned home from his doctor's appointment in follow-up to his recent hospital visit for dizziness and a subsequent fall requiring a total hip replacement. His medical history includes type 2 diabetes, decreased vision, and chronic obstructive pulmonary disease. During his prolonged hospitalization, he became depressed and forgetful. Mr. M's nurse explained to him that he needs to start taking IV antibiotics for a wound infection via a peripherally inserted central catheter line. Mr. M stared blankly and nodded that he understood. Prior to his fall, Mr. M lived alone and independently in a large house. Mr. M's frequent dizziness (a side effect of a new medication) has caused him to have a fear of falling, which subsequently generated anxiety about leaving his home to socialize with friends.

Mr. M's son is very involved in his care. Despite being well-educated, Mr. M's son became overwhelmed by the details involved in his father's at-home care and realized Mr. M needed additional support to recover from and manage his prolonged illness. He noticed that his father has difficulty understanding how to take his new medications and is taking them incorrectly. Mr. M insists to his son that he is independent and does not require any assistance.

Population Aging: The Graying of America

The world is experiencing a dramatic demographic shift. In nearly every country, the proportion of children is declining while the proportion of older adults is increasing (Uhlenberg, 2013). It is projected that by 2060, the proportion of those aged 65 and older will equal the proportion of those aged 15 and younger (Uhlenberg, 2013). The population of those 65 and older is expected to double from 35.9 to 71.5 million by 2030 (Marshall & Altpeter, 2005; Sanders, Dorfman, & Ingram, 2008).

The population of the United States is getting larger and older and these trends will reshape the nation in the coming decades. The rapid aging of the U.S. population has placed the nation in the midst of a profound demographic shift and society must address and adapt to this change (Shrestha & Heisler, 2011). Within the coming decades, one in five Americans will be eligible for Social Security and Medicare, contrasting with one in eight Americans today (Moody & Sasser, 2012).

It is estimated that by 2018, those aged 65 and older will outnumber those under the age of 5 for the first time in U.S. history. As a result, the U.S. population will look very different than ever before, representing the largest and most influential population change ever observed in American history. The sustained growth of the world's older population influences demography, economic growth, formal and informal social support systems, social insurance and pension systems, nursing practice, disease patterns, and the ability of governmental agencies to provide adequate resources. These population trends inevitably foreshadow an increased demand on health care systems. Therefore, understanding the anticipated demand and consequences of aging populations in the United States is imperative to all aspects of health care.

Definition

Population aging can be defined as: the rise in the average age of the population; an increase in the median age of the entire population; or an increase in the proportion of the population comprised by those aged 65 and older (Moody & Sasser, 2012; Shrestha & Heisler, 2011). Population aging can be explained by the demographic transition theory, which connects population change to the economic process of industrialization. Using this theory, Moody and Sasser (2012) explain that preindustrial societies often have stable populations because birth and death rates are high. Population growth occurs with industrialization because death rates often fall while birthrates remain high. Over time, birthrates are balanced with death rates and stability in population growth occurs. With the Western industrial revolution of the 19th century, a shift in the age structure of the population slowly began, known as the demographic transition. Improved agricultural production and standards of living resulted in a population with low fertility and low mortality rates. As this trend progressed, underlying drivers for population aging continued to reflect a reduction in fertility rates and increases in life expectancy as well as the post-World War II baby boom. Fast and concentrated changes in the age structure of the population were attributed, in part, to the increase in average life expectancy, the sharp decline in fertility after 1970, and mortality declines after 1950 (Moody & Sasser, 2012). This unprecedented rise in population aging created a demographic shift, often referred to as the "graying of America."

Current and Future Trends

This demographic shift encompasses a change from 1900, when only one in 25 individuals were over age 65 to a projected one in five individuals by 2030. The older population, defined as those aged 65 and older, has been increasing twice as fast as the rest of the population and is expected to represent 20.3% of the population by 2050 (Joshua & Tilly, 2002; U.S. Bureau of the Census, 2010). The population of those 65 and older has experienced a 15% increase from 35 million in 2000 to 40 million in 2010 and has risen from 3.1 million in 1900 to 40.3 million in 2010. The older population will continue to experience significant growth, especially between the years of 2010 and 2030 when the baby boom generation reaches age 65. A 36% increase is projected from 2010 to 2020 and by 2030 there is estimated to be at least 72.1 million older adults, more than twice their number in 2000.

The older population itself is increasingly older. Individuals aged 85 and older represent the fastest growing segment of the population. In 2010, those aged 65 to 74 and 75 to 84 totaled 20.8 million and 13.1 million, respectively. This number was 10 times and 17 times larger, respectively, than their numbers in 1900. In contrast, those aged 85 and older totaled 5.5 million, which was a staggering 45 times larger than their number in 1900 (Administration on Aging, 2011). The U.S. Bureau of the Census 2010 projects that by 2050, 19 million or 4.6% of the population will be age 85 and older compared to 3.1 million or 1.3% of the population in 1990 (Werner, 2011). Therefore, the older population itself is becoming increasingly older. The 65 to 74 year old age group was nearly

10 times its size in 2011 than it was in 1900, the 75 to 84 age group was 16 times larger, and the 85+ age group was a staggering 40 times larger (Administration on Aging, 2011).

It is evident that the trends of both birth and mortality and the aging of the baby boom cohorts are experiencing rapid changes. Falling birthrates and increased longevity contribute to the threat that the aging population is faced with. While this cohort continues to grow, the ratio of those aged 16 to 64 to those aged 65 and older is projected to experience a 43% decline, meaning there will be significantly fewer people to serve this rapidly growing population and provide the complex services needed (Joshua & Tilly, 2002). Hooyman (2006) stresses that no previous demographic shift will have such profound an impact on every societal institution.

Understanding the anticipated demand of aging populations in the United States and the role of the nursing profession is imperative. As the population of older individuals continues to increase in the United States, the need for appropriate care for these individuals increases as well.

Baby Boomers

The most significant and rapid population growth will occur during 2010 and 2030 when the baby boomers reach age 65. This cohort of individuals born between 1946 and 1964 is actively redefining the meaning of aging due to their cohort experiences. Born during postwar prosperity, they enjoyed tremendous opportunities in education and employment and their value systems reflect the sense of entitlement and continued economic growth they experienced. This generation includes more than 78.2 million Americans that have developed methods of coping and living that center on positivity and independence and therefore are more likely than any other cohort in history to deny or fight the aging process and to have changed the meaning of growing old (Bishop, 2009). As this cohort of older adults continues to contribute to population aging, future health care environments must work to accommodate this majority.

Health Issues

An aging population brings with it a myriad of pathologies. Glass et al. (2000) characterize that the lives of "older persons are often marked by complex changes in the capacity to function on physical, emotional, and social dimensions. These changes take place against a backdrop of profound alterations and losses in the world around them: friends and relatives die or move to institutional settings, social roles and obligations become more complex as dependence shifts, and multiple agencies may become involved in providing formal assistance" (p. 179). Aging is coupled with various changes in an individual's life, including physical, psychological, physiological, psychosocial, economic, financial, and social alterations. These changes can significantly influence the everyday lives of older persons through impacting their communication with others, perceptions of the world around them, and participation and enjoyment of activities and social interactions.

Older adults experience higher rates of comorbidities and chronic diseases coupled with less mobility and access to health care services. According to the Administration on Aging (2011), by the year 2020, 19% of older adults will have activities of daily living limitations and 4% will be severely disabled.

Chronic illness is also significantly prevalent among older adults. More than 80% of older adults suffer from at least one chronic condition (U.S. Department of Health and Human Services [USDHHS], 2010). People aged 75 and older reported an average of three chronic health problems at any given time and use an average of 4.5 prescription drugs (Berkman, Gardner, Zodikoff, & Harootyan, 2005). Chronic diseases are often coupled with disability, requiring ongoing management and unique services encompassing highly specialized medical and social care, long-term facilities, and at-home care (Berkman et al., 2005; Hooyman, 2006; Kovner, Mezey, & Harrington, 2002). Therefore, in addition to changing population demographics, this growth will influence the organization and delivery of health care due to changes in health care needs. A shift from focusing on acute disabilities and aliments to chronic diseases must occur (Berkman et al., 2005; Joshua & Tilly, 2002; Kane, 2002; Marti & Thorslund, 2007).

Furthermore, managed care and prospective payment systems have resulted in an effort to contain the costs of the growing chronically ill aging population. Patients are juggled in and out of the system and are faced with the complexity of eligibility requirements and access issues to decipher and navigate (Berkman et al., 2005).

Older adults have complex and unique biopsychological needs, diminished social status, financial hardships, and loss of family and friends (Cummings & Adler, 2007). Kane (2002) suggests that practice with older adults encompasses: addressing geriatric syndromes; attending to the functional changes accompanying chronic illness; recognizing atypical presentations of illness; and managing the multiple and simultaneous interactions of these problems. This complexity requires coordination and communication across various disciplines.

Health Literacy and Older Adults

Older adults are the fastest and largest growing segment of the U.S. population yet research has revealed they have the lowest health literacy skills when compared to other segments of the population. For the older adult population, expected to reach more than 71 million people by 2030, low health literacy can complicate already difficult health problems (USDHHS, 2010). Inadequate health literacy is therefore a significant issue for older adults. They are disproportionately affected by low health literacy because of the complexities associated with managing chronic illnesses and the changes in cognitive, physical, and sensory abilities (Speros, 2009).

Low health literacy in this growing population is associated with higher hospitalization rates, decreased use of preventive services, less knowledge about medications, increased mortality, an inability to manage chronic disease (Baker et al., 2007; Gazmarian, Williams, Peel, & Baker, 2003; Sudore et al., 2006), and lower self-reported health status (Kay & Al-Assaf, 2006). As prior research indicates, older adults utilize more health care services and have greater incidences of chronic illness compared to other segments of the population.

Managing chronic conditions requires a high level of self-care, which low health literacy significantly compromises. Older adults suffering from chronic conditions are more likely to need to navigate the health care system and understand complex health care information (USDHHS, 2010). With increases in chronic diseases due to age, older adults are exposed to making more decisions related to health care and these decisions become increasingly more complex with age (Centers for Disease Control and Prevention [CDC], 2009). Due to challenges related to physical and cognitive functioning, older adults often also have difficulties finding and using the appropriate health information (Parker, 2002).

The imperative to focus on older adults and health literacy was supported by research studies and data from the 2003 National Assessment of Adult Literacy (NAAL). The 65 years and older age group have the smallest proportion of persons with proficient health literacy skills and the highest proportion of those with below basic health literacy skills (Kutner, Greenberg, Jin, & Paulsen, 2006). The NAAL 2003 found that only 3% of older adults were determined to be proficient in health literacy and adults aged 65+ have lower health literacy scores than that of all other age groups. Specifically, 71% of adults aged 60 and older experienced difficulty in using print materials in prose form, 80% had difficulty using documents such as forms or charts, and 68% had difficulty with interpreting numbers and doing calculations (Kutner et al., 2006).

Subsequent studies have indicated that the majority of older adults in the United States lack the health literacy skills needed to utilize health-related print materials and tools with accuracy and consistency (CDC, 2009). Therefore, large segments of the population lack the basic skills necessary to make informed health care–related decisions.

In recognition of vital findings from the NAAL report related to older adults, the CDC convened an Expert Panel on Improving Health Literacy for Older Adults in 2007. This panel was designed to integrate experiences and research findings from professionals to not only assess the number of health literacy issues among the older adult population, but to identify opportunities and suggestions for health professionals to enhance the ways in which we meet the health communication needs of older adults (CDC, 2009). The goal of the panel was to enhance understanding of the scope and breadth of issues related to health literacy that affect older adults as well as brainstorm options for creating and delivering more accessible and appropriate health information to them (CDC, 2009). Conclusions indicate that while society continues to place increased demands on older adults to play an active role in their health, low health literacy acts as a significant impediment to their participation in health care activities and management (Matthews, Shine, Currie, Chan, & Kaufman, 2012).

Age-Related Challenges

While health literacy is an important, nationwide public health issue, it is clear that certain age cohorts are more at risk than others (Kay & Al-Assaf, 2006). Age-related declines and increases in the prevalence of chronic illness make older adults more susceptible to increased morbidity as a result of inadequate communication (Kay & Al-Assaf, 2006). Consequently, health disparities may arise because older adults are less able to manage their chronic illness due to a lack of understanding of health information.

Health literacy encompasses a number of cognitive processes that can pose challenges to individuals of all ages. Older adults can experience a number of changes in cognition. The three most common changes include: reduced processing speed, increased ability to become distracted, and a reduced ability to process new information. Other factors such as vision and hearing problems, stress, fatigue, depression, and medications can also reduce cognitive abilities in this population (USDHHS, 2010).

Declines in cognitive performance with age occur in more than 5 million adults aged 70 years and older in the United States (Federman, Sano, Wolf, Siu, & Halm, 2009). Sensory, perceptual, and cognitive abilities are all influenced by age. Older adults may experience declines in the speed of processing information, mental multitasking, and the ability to draw conclusions from inferences (Kay & Al-Assaf, 2006). Such thought processes involved in understanding health-related information include retrieving prescriptions and referrals, determining when to take multiple medications, comparing different insurance plans, and interpreting medical terminology.

Federman et al. (2009) aimed to study the relationship between health literacy and cognitive abilities often impaired in older adults in a cross-sectional cohort community-based sample of 414 independently living older adults. Results indicated that both memory and verbal fluency were strongly associated with health literacy, after controlling for education and health status. Health literacy was inadequate in 24.3% of the study participants. For those individuals with impaired performance on memory tests and verbal fluency, the odds of inadequate health literacy, as measured by the Short Test of Functional Health Literacy in Adults (S-TOFHLA), was three to five times those of individuals with normal cognition. The results supported the strong association between cognitive impairment and health literacy among older adults.

Similar to Ferderman et al. (2009), Speros (2009) found that as a result of declines in fluid intelligence (reasoning and processing components of learning) with age, older adults learn new information at a slower rate than younger adults. Prior research also indicates that older adults have difficulty managing multiple pieces of information at the same time (Stevens, 2003). Concepts such as "adequate," "frequently," "several times a day" can be interpreted broadly and it is therefore important to be specific with directions related to time, order, duration, and frequency. As a result, research has supported that more than 50% of all adults have challenges in comprehended instructions related to understanding their medications (Matthews et al.,

2012). Combined, these issues can make it difficult for them to not only find but use health information.

Similar to Kay and Al-Assaf (2006), Matthews et al. (2012) also aimed to establish relationships between low health literacy, health, and age. Matthews et al. (2012) sought to identify literacy-related challenges faced by older adults when managing their health and interviewed eight nurses who provided direct care to older adult populations. Thematic analysis of results from semistructured interviews identified three main themes including literacy barriers, aging process, and social resources. Results yielded multiple perspectives related to perceived challenges faced by older adults. The majority of data revealed concerns about the varying degree of health literacy among their patients and the impact it has on patients' abilities to manage their health. One of the prominent identified themes, "literacy barriers," refers to basic literacy including reading, writing, and common quantitative skills. Within the literacy barriers theme, subthemes were identified including basic literacy level, embarrassment, health literacy, minimal formal education, and numeracy. The "age-related issues" theme commonly referred to aspects such as fear of a lower quality of life as one ages, onset of health problems, isolation, dependency, acute diagnosis, and social factors. The "social resources" theme was identified as a key factor in the success of health care management strategies. Subthemes such as family support, assistance from clinicians, and community support represented different resources that can help assist the older adult in the health management process.

In addition to cognitive and sensory changes, a number or physical and psychological changes may also interfere with an older adult's ability to process health information such as changes in vision, hearing, and motor function. Considering that approximately two thirds of adults with vision problems are older than age 65, health information should be presented in an easy-to-see and read format. The font should be at least 16 to 18 points in size and it is preferable for the space between lines of text to be at least 25% of the point size. The decreased size of the pupil, a normal effect of aging, requires that older adults need more light than younger adults to see. Therefore, additional lighting is always recommended when teaching older adults. Blue colors in written text and color-coded directions should also be avoided because older adults can have difficulty distinguishing blue spectrum colors due to the yellowing of the lens with advanced age (Speros, 2009).

Since one out of three adults 60 and older have some type of hearing loss, background noise should be limited when disseminating health information to older adults. Common hearing impairments with age influence the individual's ability to discriminate between certain speech sounds. Therefore, nurses should always face the older client and ensure their face, mouth, and lips are visible to the client (Speros, 2009).

As population demographics change, standards need to be established to support and advance education of health literacy and the aging population (Kay & Al-Assaf, 2006). In order to maintain optimal health status, older adults must understand the process of effectively navigating the complex health system.

Health Literacy and the Internet

According to the U.S. Department of Commerce (2002), individuals aged 60 and older constitute the largest growing population of computer users and information seekers on the World Wide Web. Health care recipients are now empowered to get information themselves; they are expected to be informed participants in their own health care (CDC, 2009). Older adults, especially the baby boomer cohort, value ideals of independence and autonomy and they want to be in control of their own health (CDC, 2009). Therefore, an increased amount of older adults are beginning to use the Internet to access health information.

A growing body of research focuses on the social impact of the Internet, specifically its effect on health and health care. Often referred to as "e-patients," research indicates that 61% of American adults search for health information online (Fox & Jones, 2009). The Internet allows individuals to become more involved in their health care decision making by providing them access to information that was previously inaccessible. By providing older adults with health information, the Internet has the potential to empower older adults to independently manage their health and well-being (Sharit, Hernández, Czaja, & Pirolli, 2008).

However, with the burgeoning of the e-health environment, the ability of older adults to find and use e-health tools is a critical issue that warrants attention. A specific set of skills is needed to use the Internet to access health information. Obtaining information on the Internet requires knowledge of the topic of interest, basic knowledge of hardware and software operations and information seeking skills, and the ability to discern the credibility of information and its source.

Despite significant Internet use in this population, researchers have indicated that older adults often times lack the skills needed to discern the quality of the information obtained via the Internet (CDC, 2009). As individuals age, cognitive changes affect the ability to use technology. Websites often use complex technical or medical jargon, and search engines often fail to identify appropriate, accurate information. Information-seeking behavior, especially via the Internet, requires cognitive abilities such as working memory, spatial ability, and reasoning (Sharit et al., 2008). Coupled with declines in cognitive abilities with age and older adults' limited experience and knowledge with the Internet, web-based information seeking can be difficult.

A number of studies have researched how age-associated changes affect computer use. Age-related vision changes may impact an individual's ability to appropriately read a computer screen. Additionally, research details that the ability to perform certain mental operations can decrease with age, such as the ability to simultaneously remember and process new information, and comprehend text. Recent studies have focused on the emerging use of e-health tools for health information as well as the disparities in health literacy that can arise in the older populations with the advancements in technologies. Evidence indicates that many e-health tools have low effectiveness, especially for older adults (CDC, 2009).

Specifically, Sharit et al. (2008) aimed to investigate the influence of cognitive abilities on older adult information seeking on the Internet. The goal of this study was to investigate the influence of areas of Internet-related knowledge and cognitive abilities on Internet information-seeking performance by older adults. Participants were tasked with six search problems, involving information related to health and well-being. Results suggest that knowledge of certain aspects of the Internet did not fully explain information-seeking performance. Cognitive abilities significantly influenced task performance. Therefore, both Internet knowledge and key cognitive abilities were found to impact task performance. Attributes such as reasoning, working memory, and perceptual speed were all significant predictors of performance on health-related Internet search.

Fox (2005) also found that the majority of older adults are often embarrassed by their abilities to use the Internet and acknowledged a "digital divide" between older adults and other age groups. Understanding the methods in which this group obtains health information has tremendous implications on ensuring older adults obtain the health information they need, understand, and can act on.

The Internet can be an invaluable resource for older adults to empower them to become better informed about their health and health care choices, ultimately enhancing their independence and well-being. However, information seeking on the Internet requires the use of cognitive abilities and Internet experience and knowledge that older adults may lack. Unless older adults are considered in the development and implementation of advances in e-health tools, disparities among older adults will continue to increase.

As a result, the National Institute on Aging and the National Library of Medicine published a checklist that details how to make a website "senior friendly." Nurses are encouraged to provide older adults with Internet resources that are specific to older populations, such as the CDC's Health Aging web pages. In addition to "senior friendly" websites, local area agencies on aging or the Administration on Aging Eldercare Locator can help health care professional to identify local services, programs, and resources for older patients.

Promoting Health Literacy in Older Adults

As a result of disparities and gaps in access to the health care necessitating that older adults play a more active role in the management of their health, ways to facilitate their health literacy skills must be addressed (Matthews et al., 2012). Understanding the motivations and the personal and unique situations of older adults can help nurses develop and deliver effective health communication materials. Despite challenges accompanying aging, older adults have tremendous strengths that can be employed to help nurses' assist older adults with issues related to health literacy. Acknowledging these strengths and focusing on older adults' interests can empower older adults to become partners in their health and take greater control over their health decisions (USDHHS, 2010).

Age-appropriate teaching strategies for older adults must be planned and purposeful, and adapted to accommodate the specific needs of each individual (Speros, 2009). Speros (2009) identifies strategies that should be an intimate part of nurses' teaching repertoire to promote health literacy. These strategies center on a model of teaching older adults called geragogy. This framework establishes teaching interventions that compensate for the cognitive, sensory, and physical effects of aging while fostering independences (Speros, 2009). Such age-appropriate teaching strategies include approaching the older adults in a manner that facilities respect, acceptance, and support and allowing time to process new information. Teaching sessions should ideally be scheduled in the mid-morning and long, lengthy sessions should be avoided. New knowledge or skills should be linked to past experiences to help older adults reconnect with lived experiences to facilitate learning. Creating a shame-free environment and emphasizing the importance of understanding will encourage older adults to remain active partners in their health care. Learning should always emphasize maintenance of independence and practicality while keeping the content relevant to their daily activities, social structure, and physical function. Nurses should employ teaching that is slow and deliberate, allowing the older adult to establish a personal timeline for learning (Speros, 2009). Directions should be provided in concrete terms that engage participation during teaching and essential points should be repeated frequently throughout the teaching session.

A "Universal Precaution" approach can also be used to educate patients. This approach encourages providers to teach all their patients using simple, plain language (Cutilli & Schaefer, 2011). Several methods that are useful in providing effective health education include the use of teach-back, multimedia material including visual aids, plain language, appropriate medical terminology and supporting a person's life experiences. Additionally, the CDC (2011) has outlined key points to consider when designing health materials for older adults such as making the information personal, empowering, self-directed, and solution-oriented. Nurses should provide older adults with information they can relate to that shows respect for their background and values. Framing the material in a manner that will enable older adults to feel confident they can take control over their own health will allow them to feel they can use this information to impact their lives. Additionally, nurses should provide a short, concise health message with specific action steps that detail how to achieve the specific desired health goal.

Nurses can implement these age-appropriate teaching strategies in order to improve the health literacy of an aging patient. In addition to these communication techniques, nurses can observe subtle cues suggesting low health literacy, such as not having reading glasses available, displaying unusually angry behavior when asked to complete forms, or asking to review information with a significant other before making a health care decisions (American Medical Association, 2007, as cited in Cutilli & Schaefer, 2011). Such strategies, when employed, can enhance communication with older adults.

Implications to Nursing Practice

Low health literacy among older adults presents a challenge to not only patients but health care providers as well (Cutilli & Schaefer, 2011). Health care professionals have an obligation to teach their patients effectively. Patient education is a core responsibility of the nursing profession. However, many nurses and other health care professionals have not been appropriately trained to iden-tify and interact with patients with low health literacy (Sand-Jecklin, Marray, Summers, & Watson, 2010).

Sand-Jecklin et al. (2010) stress that all nurses and nursing students must be able to assess patients for health literacy limitations and ensure patients' understanding of important health information. It is an imperative for health literacy–related content to be incorporated into nursing education curricula to make certain new nurses are skilled in communicating with patients with low health literacy (Sand-Jecklin et al., 2010).

Sand-Jecklin et al. (2010) conducted an exploratory study to evaluate the impact of a health literacy education session on student knowledge. Results indicated that there was a significant increase in nursing student knowledge scores following the education session. Despite significant implications for nursing practice and education, the study failed to identify whether students continue to retain and use the knowledge gained through this session.

Because age-related changes pose significant challenges in communicating with older adults, nurses must be proactive in promoting clear communication that is both individualized and increases comprehension. Speros (2009) stresses that nurses have a professional, ethical, and legal responsibility to communi-cate health information to older adults in a way in which they can understand. However, nurses may lack the knowledge and skills needed to appropriately meet the learning and communication needs of elderly patients.

Summary

An understanding of the impact of health literacy on health outcomes is essen-tial for providing effective care for older adults. A population of over 71.5 mil-lion adults aged 65 and older by 2030, combined with results from the NAAL report, substantiate the imperative to improve the delivery of health informa-tion to older adults. Promoting health literacy in older adults has been identi-fied as a public health imperative. Low health literacy in the United States is costly in terms of poor health outcomes as well as the financial burden it places on health care systems (Sand-Jecklin et al., 2010). Estimates total approximately $73 billion in unnecessary health care costs as a result of low health literacy through misunderstanding of health information and subsequent patient non-compliance (Center for Health Care Strategies, 2000 as cited in Speros, 2009).

Research over the last decade consistently demonstrates that older adults have higher rates of low health literacy compared to the rest of the population. It is evident that older adults comprise a unique subset of the population with a diverse set of needs and preferences. They have more chronic illnesses and utilized more medical services than any other cohort of the U.S. population. Variations in access to information, the complexity of health information, and normal age-related changes can compromise an older adult's ability to use and make sense of health information (CDC, 2011).

Research findings support the imperative to increase awareness and establish standards and protocols to communicate with individuals aged 65 years and older. Matthews et al. (2012) concludes that research findings strongly support the need to develop an "elder communication protocol" to address these barriers and risk factors, in order to decrease health disparities and ultimately improve the health care quality for this growing population.

Research must continue to work to identify gaps related to older adults and health literacy and create opportunities for health professionals to better meet the health and communication needs of this population. Future research endeavors must establish ways to help adults effectively navigate and utilize the health care system and health information. It is of vital importance that researchers develop a concrete understanding of the determinants of limited health literacy in aging and at what point these declines begin. Such findings will enable development of specific approaches to address health literacy disparities in older adults (CDC, 2009).

In order to consistently and appropriately manage their health and prevent disease, health information to older adults must be disseminated in a health literate manner. Aspects of health literacy must be addressed in order to attenuate the health disparities arising in this population (Kay & Al-Assaf, 2006).

References

Administration on Aging. (2011). *A profile of older Americans: 2012, Administration on Aging.* Retrieved from http://www.aoa.gov/Aging_Statistics/Profile/index.aspx

American Medical Association. (2007). *Health literacy and patient safety: Help your patients understand. Manual for clinicians* (2nd ed.). Chicago, IL: American Medical Association and American Medical Foundation.

Baker, D. W., Wolf, M. S., Feinglass, J., Thompson, J. A., Gazmararian, J. A., & Huang, J. (2007). Health literacy and mortality among elderly persons. *Archive of Internal Medicine, 167*(14), 1503–1509.

Berkman, B. J., Gardner, D. S., Zodikoff, B. D., & Harootyan, L. K. (2005). Social work in health care with older adults: Future challenges. *Families in Society: The Journal of Contemporary Social Services, 86*(3), 329–337.

Bishop, J. A. (2009). *Booming towards aging in place: The 21st century specialization for interior designers.* Retrieved from http://www.bishopinteriors.com/BDG/images/Bishop_J-Booming_Towards_Aging_in_Place-rev4.pdf

Center for Health Care Strategies. (2000). CHCS fact sheet. *Facts about health literacy: Low health literacy skills increase annual health care expenditures by $73 billion.* Princeton, NJ: Center for Health Care Strategies.

Centers for Disease Control and Prevention. (2009). *Improving health literacy for older adults: Expert panel report 2009.* Atlanta, GA: U.S. Department of Health and Human Services.

Centers for Disease Control and Prevention. (2011). *Older adults: How do older adults make decisions?* Retrieved from http://www.cdc.gov/healthliteracy/developmaterials/audiences/olderadults/understanding-decisions.html

Cummings, S., & Adler, G. (2007). Predictors of social workers employment in gerontological work. *Educational Gerontology, 33,* 925–938.

Cutilli, C. C., & Schaefer, C. T. (2011). Case studies in geriatric health literacy. *Orthopaedic Nursing, 30*(4), 281–285.

Federman, A. D., Sano, M., Wolf, M. S., Siu, A. L., & Halm, E. A. (2009). Health literacy and cognitive performance in older adults. *Journal of the American Geriatrics Society, 57,* 1475–1490.

Fox, S. (2005). *Digital divisions.* Washington, DC: Pew Internet & American Life Project. Retrieved from http://www.pewinternet.org/Reports/2005/DigitalDivisions.aspx

Fox, S., & Jones, S. (2009). *The social life of health information.* Washington, DC: Pew Internet & American Life Project.

Gazmarian, J. A., William, M. V., Peel, J., & Baker, D. W. (2003). Health literacy and knowledge of chronic disease. *Patient Education and Counseling, 51,* 267–275.

Glass, T., Dym, B., Greenberg, S., Rintell, D., Roesch, C., & Berkman, L. (2000). Psychosocial intervention in stroke: Families in Recovery From Stroke Trial (FIRST). *American Journal of Orthopsychiatry, 70*(2), 169–181.

Hooyman, N. (2006). *Achieving curricular and organizational change: Impact of the CSWE Geriatric Enrichment in Social Work Education Project.* Alexandria, VA: Council on Social Work Education.

Joshua, M. W., & Tilly, J. (2002). Population ageing in the United States of America: Implications for public programmes. *International Journal of Epidemiology, 31*(4), 776–781.

Kane, R. L. (2002). The future history of geriatrics: Geriatrics at the crossroads. *Journal of Gerontology, 57A*(12), M803–M805.

Kay, T. L., & Al-Assaf, A. (2006, Fall). *Health literacy: Impact on older adults.* AAMA executive. Chicago, IL: American Academy of Medical Administrators.

Kovner, C. T., Mezey, M., & Harrington, C. (2002). Who care for older adults? Workforce implications of an aging society. *Health Affairs, 21*(5), 78–89.

Kutner, M., Greenberg, E., Jin, Y., & Paulsen, C. (2006). *The health literacy of America's adults: Results from the 2003 National Assessment of Adult Literacy.* Washington, DC: U.S. Government Printing Office. Retrieved from http://nces.ed.gov/pubsearch/pubsinfo.asp?pubid=2006483

Marshall, V. W., & Altpeter, M. (2005). Cultivating social work leadership in health promotion and aging: Strategies for active aging interventions. *Health and Social Work, 30*(2), 135–145.

Marti, G. P., & Thorslund, M. (2007). Health trends in the elderly population: Getting better and getting worse. *The Gerontologist, 47*(2), 150–158.

Matthews, L. A., Shine, A. L., Currie, L., Chan, C. V., & Kaufman, D. R. (2012). *A nurse's eye-view on health literacy in older adults.* Proceedings from the 11th International Congress on Nursing Informatics, Montreal, Canada.

Moody, H. R., & Sasser, J. R. (2012). *Aging: Concepts and controversies* (7th ed.). Thousand Oaks, CA: Pine Forge Press.

Parker, R. (2002). Health literacy: A challenge for American patients and their health care providers. *Health Promotion International, 14*(4), 277–283.

Sanders, S., Dorfman, L., & Ingram, J. (2008). An evaluation of the GeroRich program for infusing social work curriculum with aging content. *Gerontology & Geriatric Education, 28*(4), 22–38.

Sand-Jecklin, K., Murray, B., Summers, B., & Watson, J. (2010). Educating nursing students about health literacy: From the classroom to the patient bedside. *The Online Journal of Issues in Nursing, 1*(3).

Sharit, J., Hernández, M. A., Czaja, S. J., & Pirolli, P. (2008). Investigating the roles of knowledge and cognitive abilities in older adult information seeking on the web. *Transactions of Computer-Human Interaction, 15*, 11–25.

Shrestha, L., & Heisler, E. (2011). The changing demographic profile of the United States [PDF document]. *Federation of American Scientists.* Retrieved from http://www.fas.org

Speros, C. I. (2009). More than words: Promoting health literacy in older adults. *The Online Journal of Issues in Nursing, 14*(3).

Stevens, B. (2003). *How seniors learn.* Issue Brief. Center for Medicare Education, *4*(9). Retrieved from http://www.mathematica-mpr.com/PDFs/howseniors.pdf

Sudore, R. L., Yaffe, K., Satterfield, S., Harris, T. B., Mehta, K. M., Simonsick, E. M., & Schillinger, D. (2006). Limited literacy and mortality in the elderly: The health, aging, and body composition study. *Journal of General Internal Medicine, 21*, 806–812.

Uhlenberg, P. (2013, Spring). Demography is not destiny: The challenges and opportunities of global population aging. *Generations: Journal of the American Society on Aging, 37*(1), 12–18.

U.S. Census Bureau. (2010). Decennial census of population, 1900 to 2000. *Census Summary File 1.* Washington, DC.

U.S. Department of Commerce. (2002). *A nation online: How Americans are expanding their use of the internet.* Washington, DC: NTIA and the Economics and Statistics Administration.

U.S. Department of Health and Human Services. Office of Disease Prevention and Health Promotion. (2010). *Quick guide to health literacy and older adults.* Retrieved from http://www.health.gov/communication/literacy/olderadults/literacy.htm

Werner, C. A. (2011). *The older population: 2010, 2010 census briefs.* Retrieved from http://www.census.gov/prod/cen2010/briefs/c2010br-09.pdf

Research Participants

Hallie Kassan

Case Scenario

A physician researcher would like to collect data on the outcomes of patients in his practice who undergo surgical procedures for a spine condition. The information that the researcher wants to collect is important, as it can lead to more knowledge about how to manage pain and improve functionality after these surgeries. The study will be conducted by distributing surveys through the mail to patients who have undergone this procedure. To determine which patients have undergone the procedure, ICD-10 codes in the medical record are reviewed. Shortly after sending out the targeted surveys, the Institutional Review Board (IRB), the group charged with protection of human research subjects, begins receiving phone calls from potential research participants. Upon further phone conversation, it is revealed by each potential research participant that the stated procedure was never had. Upon a collaborative review of the medical record it was determined by the investigator and IRB that all potential participants actually did undergo the procedure. Because these potential research participants were not aware of the procedure they underwent, the survey was not completed. As a result, the researcher will be limited in the amount of data he is able to collect.

In another research study, a physician researcher would like to see if taking one dose of an investigational drug in the morning and one dose in the evening reduces the incidence of heart attack in a diabetic population. Some of the participants in the study do not understand the directions for taking the medication. Rather than taking one dose of the drug in the morning and one dose again in the evening, they take two doses of the drug at the same time. Incorrectly taking an investigational drug places these research participants at a greater risk for adverse effects. This error also has an adverse impact on the scientific integrity of the data. If participants are not able to comply with the study medication regimen, the researcher will not know whether the drug regimen had an effect on incidences of heart attack. Furthermore, when the scientific integrity of data is affected, research participants are placed at greater risk.

Research Participants and Health Literacy—The Problem

These case scenarios are representative of the potential impact of low health literacy on human subjects research. As suggested in the 2004 Institute of Medicine (IOM) report, health literacy skills are needed for a person to make a decision about participating in a research study (Nielsen-Bohlman, Panzer, & Kindig, 2004). While health literacy skills are important for making that initial decision, they are also important throughout participation in a research study.

Human subjects research is defined as a systematic investigation designed to contribute to generalizable knowledge in which a researcher obtains data through intervention or interaction with a living individual (Protection of Human Subjects, 45 CFR 46, 1991). Human subjects research, also known as clinical trials or clinical research, is essential to advancing the fields of medicine and science. Without research, new treatments and interventions cannot be discovered, diseases cannot be cured, and information about the safety and efficacy of new therapies cannot be learned. Thus, research participants are valuable resources to the health care community and should be protected.

When conducting human subjects research, researchers need to adhere to the Belmont Report. The Belmont Report outlines three ethical principles of human subjects research: Respect for Persons, Beneficence, and Justice (Belmont Report, 1979). All three principles of the Belmont Report correlate with the need to ensure that research participants with low health literacy are protected.

Respect for Persons

The first principle, respect for persons, discusses the idea that research participants must be considered autonomous individuals (Belmont Report, 1979). They should be allowed to make their own independent choice about participating in a research study by being fully informed about what they are agreeing to do. In addition, vulnerable populations may need extra protections. This can be accomplished through an informed consent process.

Federal regulations require informed consent to be obtained and documented before a person can participate in a research study. IRBs review and approve all informed consent documents before they can be used in a research study. Research has been done to try to understand whether or not consent for a research study is truly informed. In a study that looked at the quality of consent in a cancer clinical trial, it was found that although 90% of the participants were satisfied with the informed consent process, many did not understand particular features of the trials, such as the investigational nature of the treatment (Joffe, Cook, Cleary, Clark, & Weeks, 2001). Other research has shown that only 28% of research participants understand the research study after one pass through a consent form (Sudore et al., 2006). If a person does not fully comprehend participation in a research study, withdrawal from the study before it concludes is more likely (Stryker, Wray, Emmons, Winer, & Demetri, 2006).

Researchers focus heavily on the informed consent document. However, studies have shown that in addition to the consent document, other methods are needed to truly obtain an informed consent. Whether the consent is concise or long, there tends to be no statistically significant difference in the research participants comprehension of the document (Enama et al., 2012). This suggests the need for other methods to obtain informed consent for research participation.

Beneficence

The second principle of the Belmont Report, the principle of beneficence, focuses on research maximizing benefit and minimizing risk and researchers doing no harm (Belmont Report, 1979). A person's risk in participating in research is reduced when they can truly comprehend the research study.

As in standard care, research studies often require medications to be taken at certain times or with certain types of foods. In addition, certain approved medications may be prohibited from being taken with an investigational medication received as part of a research study. In 2007, Wolf et al. performed a study in which patients were shown prescription pill containers and asked questions to assess their understanding of the medication instructions. In this study, 46% of patients did not understand one or more dosage instructions. If patients cannot understand medication instructions as part of regular medical care, they will have the same problems when enrolled in a research study. In addition, since research treatments tend to be investigational, noncompliance or erroneous dosing may subject a research participant to a risk that is unknown. Finally, as depicted in the case scenario, when research participants are noncompliant or take erroneous doses of medication, it impacts upon patient safety and patient outcomes, as well as the scientific validity of the data. Thus, not only is the specific participant at risk, but all participants become exposed to a greater risk. If valid data cannot be obtained from a research study, then all participants were placed at risk, by virtue of their participation, by a study which may not achieve any results.

In addition to being able to understand dosing of medications, research participants need to show up for study visits and report any adverse events they experience. People with low health literacy may not be able read appointment slips or understand that any side effects experienced should be explained to the researcher (Nielsen-Bohlman et al., 2004). Again, these are skills necessary to minimize risk and maximize the benefits of research. Neglecting to convey side effects can put others in the research study at risk if important risks are being overlooked. Finally, missing a scheduled study visit can put the individual research participant at risk if the researcher is not able to ensure, with an in-person visit, that the participant is not being adversely effected by the research study.

Justice

The third principle of the Belmont Report is the principle of justice. Health literacy is an important consideration in this principle as well. Justice requires that the risks and benefits of human subjects research be distributed across all populations, races, and ethnicities (Belmont Report, 1979). Thus, if one population is less health literate than another, there may unequal representation of those populations in research studies.

An IOM report from 2003 indicated that racial and ethnic health disparities exist across many diseases (Smedly, Stith, & Nelson, 2003). Early death and increased burden of disease have been found to pervade health-disparate populations (Nolte & McKee, 2008). Thus, it is important for these minority populations to enroll in research studies. However, according to a Food and Drug Administration (FDA) review, African Americans, Asian/Pacific Islanders, Hispanic/Latinos, and Native Americans collectively represented less than 10% of participants in clinical trials for cancer drugs in 1995 to 1999 (Evelyn et al., 2001), and this is a type of statistic not exclusive to cancer research. The complexity of consent forms and research study materials has been cited as a potential barrier to participation in research for these groups of people (Killien et al., 2000).

When a population is unequally represented in a research study, the results of the study may not be applicable and useful in that population. In addition, results of research studies are less generalizable when populations are underrepresented. One cannot infer the efficacy and safety of a drug in a demographic population that is not part of the research study. Different races and ethnicities have different genetic makeups that can cause reactions to drugs that were not discovered in the population that participated in the research study to examine the drug. New side effects may appear or a drug may not be as effective in a person of a different demographic. Thus, it is important to address the issue of comprehension and consent when enrolling participants into clinical studies and ensure that those with all levels of health literacy participate.

Significance

Participating in a research study may be part of the decision a person needs to make regarding his or her health. Giving consent for participation in research requires a level of comprehension above that of consent for medical care. For certain conditions, a clinical study offers a course of treatment. Even if participation in a research study does not offer a course of treatment, it allows an individual to contribute to the medical field and help to advance science. Without research participants, the field of medicine could not move forward.

In addition, regulations governing human subjects research designate certain categories of research participants as vulnerable. Participants considered vulnerable are those who may require extra protections when participating in research studies. Specifically, the regulations designate children, pregnant women, prisoners, and the decisionally impaired as vulnerable (Protection of Human Subjects, 45 CFR 46, 1991). However, persons with low health literacy are not designated as a vulnerable population requiring additional protections. Thus, it is important for researchers to be aware of a person's health literacy skills. Even if regulations do not specifically call for it, researchers should use additional safeguards to ensure that those who participate in research and have low health literacy are adequately protected.

In order to ensure that all three ethical principles of the Belmont Report are being met when conducting research, it is important for researchers to consider the tools and assistance they can provide those research subjects with low health literacy.

Implications to Nursing Practice

Nurses can play an important role in conducting human subjects research. Nurses often serve as research managers or research coordinators for individual studies. As managers or coordinators, they will have the most contact with research participants.

Throughout the conduct of a research study, there are many strategies that can be employed to assist subjects with low health literacy gain a better understanding of research participation. Strategies should be used beginning with the creation of the study documents, including the consent form, and continuing throughout a research participant's study participation. As discussed earlier, protecting and assisting those with low health literacy are essential for maintaining the principles of the Belmont Report.

Respect for Persons and Beneficence

All human subjects research studies require review and approval by an IRB before research participants can be enrolled. Once a research study is approved by an IRB, researchers can begin recruitment. One step to protect those with limited health literacy is ensuring an adequate consent process, which encompasses the document and the discussion.

IRBs need to review and approved the informed consent document that will be used for the research study. According to federal regulations, consent forms need to be written "in language understandable to the subject" (Protection of Human Subjects, 45 CFR 46, 1991). In addition, the International Conference on Harmonization Guidelines, which are followed by those who conduct research, state, "The language used in the oral and written information about the trial, including the written informed consent form, should be as nontechnical as practical and should be understandable to the subject. . . ." (International Conference on Harmonization–Guidelines for Good Clinical Practice, 1996). Finally, the IOM Report, *Health Literacy: A Prescription to End Confusion,* found that the readability level of research consent forms exceed the average reading level of adults in the United States (Nielsen-Bohlman et al., 2004). Therefore, nurses should ensure that consent forms submitted to the IRB for review and approval are written in plain language and are action oriented and as understandable as possible. This can be done by following suggestions outlined in the Program for Readability in Science & Medicine (PRISM) readability toolkit (Ridpath, Greene, & Wiese, 2007). Using techniques such as plain language, serif fonts, pictures, and left justification when creating a consent form can contribute to a research participant's ability to read and comprehend the information in a consent form. During a literature review, Houts, Doak, Doak, and Loscalzo (2006) found that illustrations can improve attention, comprehension, recall, and adherence to health-related information. This concept of illustrations can also be applied to research consent forms. Although the written consent form is only the written document and assists in the consent process, having an understandable consent document can greatly assist in the research participant's ability to comprehend the research.

Studies have been done to see if a simplified or shortened consent form can improve comprehension during the consent process. In one study, subjects were randomized to standard consent documents or consent documents that were modified to be easy to read (Coyne et al., 2003). The easy-to-read consent statements made changes including, but not limited to, text style, font, and vocabulary. The study found that subjects who were consented with the easy-to-read consent document did not have a greater comprehension of the study than those consented with the standard document. Although ensuring the readability of a consent document is important to assist with comprehension, other safeguards are also needed to ensure protection of all potential research participants.

Obtaining true informed consent for participation in research is the responsibility of the researcher, not of the research participant. Researchers should always keep in mind that informed consent is a process and the document should enhance and reinforce the conversation about the study. Although the regulations governing human subjects research (Protection of Human Subjects, 45 CFR 46, 1991) specifically cite the use of a document, researchers should make sure to put thought into the entire process.

The consent process begins at the time of recruitment. Research participants have to truly understand that they are agreeing to participate in a research study, which is designed to generate new scientific knowledge. Depending on the research study, a participant may or may not benefit from participation. In addition, even if there is a chance of benefit, it is never guaranteed. Each of these concepts can be difficult to comprehend.

As commented on by Schenker and Meisel (2011), the timing of a consent process can improve comprehension. Although their commentary related to informed consent for clinical care, their thoughts can be applied to research studies. If a researcher wants to approach someone to participate in a research study, providing participants more time to contemplate the risks and benefits of their participation can aid in the complete comprehension of the study participation. Suggested methods to provide the additional time include: (1) providing potential participants with the opportunity to review the consent form and come back at a later time to complete the consent process and sign the document, (2) mailing the consent document in advance of scheduled appointment time, and (3) scheduling screening visits that allow for an adequate amount of time to discuss the research study.

Researchers should ensure that they allow adequate time for consenting research participants. Consenting in an atmosphere that does not feel rushed can help ensure a research participant's comprehension, and thus add to minimization of risks. Researchers should avoid consent for a research study during times of stress or anxiety, such as immediately after a person receives a new or life-threatening diagnosis or when a person is being prepared for a major surgery.

Potential research participants should be encouraged to bring additional support people with them, such as friends or relatives (Jefford & Moore, 2008). After the in-person consent discussion occurs, a follow-up telephone conversation with a nurse involved in the research has been found to be helpful in improving potential research participants' awareness and understanding of research studies (Aaronson et al., 1996).

Researchers can also use additional alternative methods during the consent process. In the new era of technology, researchers can consider using visual aid technology during the consent process in addition to the consent form. Types of technology that can be used include tablets, computers, and videos. A literature review was recently done to look at the studies that have examined consent processes that include the use of multimedia aids (Palmer, Lanouette, & Jeste, 2012). Of the studies reviewed, 50% found those that took part in multimedia-aided consent had a significantly enhanced understanding of the information provided than those who did not have the multimedia aid. However, additional research is needed to determine which types of multimedia tools are best in specific contexts or with specific populations (Palmer, Lanouette, & Jeste, 2012).

An example of how technology can be integrated into the consent process was examined by Rowbotham et al. with the use of iPads (Rowbotham, Astin, Greene, & Cummings, 2013). Research participants who were randomized to the interactive tablet consent or a standard consent process. Those randomized to the interactive tablet consent listened to an information video at the beginning of the consent process and then completed a quiz at the end of the consent process. The quiz was meant to assess their comprehension about participation in the research study. When completing the quiz, if participants marked an answer wrong, the tablet would return back to the section of the consent form that was relevant to that question. The study found that participants who had been consented with a tablet were more likely to answer the questions correctly on a follow-up survey regarding the research study, than participants who had gone through the standard consent process. This study not only highlights the usefulness of a tablet during a consent process, but also highlights the importance of comprehension assessment.

A comprehension assessment should be done before a research participant signs the consent document. This assessment is part of the consent process. The assessment can be done by the use of a quiz at the end of the consent form (Figure 15.1) or by incorporating a variation of the teach-back method (Figure 15.2).

Using a teach-back method can be more challenging for the researcher as he or she must be familiar with the process, and realize that when done correctly, it involves more than asking yes or no questions. When researchers plan to use the teach-back method when obtaining consent, it is helpful to participate in training beforehand. Training can consist of practice consent form sessions, where the researcher practices consenting a mock research subject. In addition, the questions the researchers should ask the subjects can be incorporated into the researcher's version of the consent form. Using a consent form with tips and questions on it can assist the researcher through the consent process, and ensure that questions are asked of the research participant at the correct time (Koziatek & Young, 2012).

In addition, a teach-to-goal strategy (Paasche-Orlow, 2005) can be employed during the consent process. When using teach-to-goal, researchers should continue to provide education about the research to the research participant until the participant has a complete understanding of the study. Researchers should ask participants questions about the research study at the end of the consent process. If the participant does not answer the question correctly, the researcher should educate the participant. After the education, the researcher should again see if the participant can answer questions correctly. This cycle should be repeated until answers to all questions are correct. One study, using a teach-to-goal strategy, eventually achieved comprehension in 98% of participants (Sudore et al., 2006).

Research Review Questionnaire:

After reviewing the consent form for this study please answer the following questions by circling "True" <u>or</u> "False." The researchers doing this study want to be sure that you know what is involved in being in this research study. This questionnaire will help them make that decision. You may ask questions of the researcher and review the consent form again at any time.

- I am being asked to be in a research study.
    True   False

- This study involves the use of MRIs and neurocognitive testing.
    True   False

- I have to participate in this research study to receive care.
    True   False

- I can withdraw from participating in this study at any time.
    True   False

- There are no potential risks or discomforts to me from participating.
    True   False

- I am guaranteed to feel better from being in this study.
    True   False

<u>**For research staff only**</u>
Notes concerning research review questionnaire:

_____
_____
_____

Figure 15.1 Sample Research Review Questionnaire.

Comprehensive Assessment Form

Subject Name/Initials: _____ Evaluation Date: _____

Directions for the evaluator:
Make a subjective judgment regarding item 1. Ask the subject questions 2 to 6 and record responses. You may use different wording to assist in enhancing the subject's understanding of the question.

1. Is the subject alert and able to communicate with you?   Yes   No

2. Ask the subject if he or she understands that he or she is being asked to be in a research study. Ask the subject to describe in his or her own words how the study activities or treatment differs from his or her regular care.

    _____

    _____

    _____

3. Ask the subject to name at least two potential risks of being in the study. _____

    _____

4. Ask the subject to name at least two things that he or she will be expected to do during the study._____

5. Ask the subject to explain what he or she would do if he or she no longer wanted to be in the study._____

6. Ask the subject to explain what he or she would do if he or she experienced distress or discomfort during the study. _____

Evaluators Statement: In my opinion, the subject is alert, able to communicate, and has provided acceptable answers to the questions above.

Evaluators Signature:_____ Date:_____

Figure 15.2 Comprehensive Assessment Form.

Educational sessions have also been found to help improve research subjects' comprehension of research studies. Wallace, Fleshner, Jewett, Basiuk, and Crook (2006) explored the idea of offering educational sessions about a research study before participants sign consent forms. The educational sessions consisted of a video, presentation from a clinical trial participant about his opinion on clinical trials and a presentation from physicians involved in the study. Potential research participants attended the sessions before meeting individually with their clinician. In addition, they were encouraged to bring a partner to the session. This way, they would have someone with whom to discuss research study participation. They found that the educational sessions assisted potential subjects in making an informed decision about whether or not to participate in the research study and increased accrual into the study (Wallace et al., 2006). This is another method that research nurses can incorporate to attempt to improve comprehension and provide additional safeguards to research participants with low health literacy.

Informed decision aids may also assist in the decision-making process for joining research studies. Decision aids are "interventions designed to help people make specific deliberative choices among options by providing information on the options and outcomes relevant to a patient's health" (O'Connor et al., 1999). Decision aids improve patients' knowledge about options, while reducing their decisional conflict in the clinical care setting (O'Connor et al., 1999). Based on this information, a study was done to look at the usefulness of decision aids in a research study. The decision aid used in this study contained diagrams, graphics, and personalized worksheets to help potential research participants weigh the pros and cons of participation in a research study (Juraskova et al., 2008). Results of this study showed that use of the decision aid assisted research participants in understanding the study, as more than 80% of items on a survey were answered correctly.

Achieving true informed consent is the first step in protecting all research participants and especially those with low health literacy. Once consent is achieved, researchers should have ongoing one-on-one discussions with participants at study visits. Although the consent form has already been signed, researchers should use teach-to-goal methods throughout the study to ensure continued understanding of participation and directions that need to be followed. When medication is prescribed as part of a research study, researchers need to ensure that research participants understand how to take those medications. It was found that health care providers, in the clinical care setting, are not adequately communicating instructions for taking medications to patients (Hernandez, 2008). Researchers need to be even more careful about ensuring research participants understand how to comply with investigational medications. They can do this by using the teach-back method and using pill compliance diaries. Participants can be instructed to bring the diaries with them to each study visit. Reviewing the diaries at research study visits will provide the researcher with an understanding as to whether or not the participant is compliant with the medication regimen.

Justice

As indicated earlier, in order to ensure that there is equitable selection of participants in research studies, provisions should be made to address issues of low health literacy in minority populations. In addition to the principle of justice (Belmont Report, 1979), the NIH Revitalization Act of 1993 indicated that researchers must ensure that minorities are represented in clinical trials (U.S. Department of Health and Human Services, 2003). Without equal representation across all groups, risks and benefits are not equally distributed and the generalizability of results is reduced. Lack of time spent by researchers discussing potential risks of research studies and lack of clinicians and patient advocates who speak the language of the potential participants have been found to be potential barriers to participation in research studies (Ford et al., 2013). In addition, African Americans have specifically cited lack of understanding of the consent, due to medical and legal terminology as a barrier to participation in research studies (Corbie-Smith, Thomas, Williams, & Moody-Ayers, 1991).

Discussions about increasing minority enrollment into research studies always focus on increasing a potential research participant's understanding of the research study and the general importance of research. Thus, when enrolling minority subjects who may have low health literacy into research studies, researchers should ensure that extra time is allotted to the consent process. They should allow potential participants to have sufficient time to consider their options and potentially receive additional viewpoints from places such as the library or from family and friends (Corbie-Smith et al., 1991). Partnering with community organizations in the areas in which minorities will be recruited can also help to access and protect potential research participants. Representatives from community organizations tend to be of the same race and ethnicity and come from similar life experiences. The community representatives may be helpful in overcoming some of the health literacy barriers by bridging the gap between physicians and potential research participants (Alvarez, Vasquez, Mayorga, Feaster, & Mitrani, 2006).

In addition, community representatives know the language that the potential research participant speaks and can serve as advocates and ensure that someone is available who speaks the participants preferred language. This can be accomplished through in-person interpreters or telephonic interpreters, if no one is available in person. Putting these additional safeguards in place may help facilitate participation of minorities, and in turn increase generalizability of the results.

If a researcher knows that a population with low health literacy will be a target of the research or the population could benefit from the research, it would be helpful for the researcher to engage a health literacy advisory group to assist with the implementation of the study (Schillinger & Keller, 2011). Using a health literacy advisory group can help create study materials and communication strategies that are understandable to the research participant population. This could result in an increase in participation of individuals with low health literacy.

Summary

When serving as researchers, nurses should be aware of the impact that low health literacy may have on research participation as well as the outcomes of research studies. Through education, issues of health literacy and its impact on clinical research should be communicated to all researchers.

It is important to apply additional safeguards for those with low health literacy when doing human subjects research in order to uphold the principles of the Belmont Report: Respect for Persons, Beneficence, and Justice. There are different approaches that can be used throughout the conduct of a research study to ensure these principles are being upheld.

Providing additional safeguards also improves the chances of obtaining valuable results. Ensuring that research participants are well informed and understand study procedures and protocol compliance increases the probability that a study will be successful. This ensures that participants are not subjected to unnecessary additional risk.

Persons with low health literacy do not always stand out. It may not be obvious to a researcher that someone has low health literacy. Thus, it is important to consider applying the additional protections, discussed in this chapter, to all research participants.

Conducting human subjects research entails following many policies and regulations. Because of this, implementing additional safeguards may seem burdensome. Hopefully, nurse researchers can understand that it is ultimately in their best interests to ensure the protection of those with low health literacy.

Finally, it is important to note that the suggestions presented in this chapter are not specific to research studies. Most of the suggested practices can and may be implemented during the course of all clinical care.

Research is an important area of medicine as it provides a basis for evidence-based medicine. Nurse researchers serve important roles in the conduct of research, as they are often the researchers having the most participant contact. Currently health care is moving toward a more patient-centered model. Patient-centered models focus on the patient taking a more active role in his or her own care. Research should move toward the same, a research-participant centered model. A research-participant centered model for research would serve well in upholding the three ethical principles of the Belmont Report. The importance of the nurse–patient partnership in the patient-centered model has been explored by Doss, DePascal, and Hadley (2011). Nurses can form the same types of partnerships with research subjects, allowing research participants to take a more active role in decisions about research participation. Using some of the techniques described in this chapter can assist in forming those partnerships and overcome some of the barriers of low health literacy.

References

Aaronson, N. K., Visser-Pol, E., Leenhouts, G. H., Muller, M. J., van der Schot, A. C., van Dam, F. S., . . . Dubbelman, R. (1996). Telephone-based nursing intervention improves the effectiveness of the informed consent process in cancer clinical trials. *Journal of Clinical Oncology, 14*(3), 984–996.

Alvarez, R. A., Vasquez, E., Mayorga, C. C., Feaster, D. J., & Mitrani, V. B. (2006). Increasing minority research participation through community organization outreach. *Western Journal of Nursing Research, 28*(5), 541–563.

Corbie-Smith, G., Thomas, S. B., Williams, M. V., & Moody-Ayers, S. (1991). Attitudes and beliefs of African Americans toward participation in medical research. *Journal of Internal Medicine, 14*, 537–546.

Coyne, C. A., Xu, R., Raich, P., Plomer, K., Dignan, M., Wenzel, L. B., . . . Cella, D., & Eastern Cooperative Oncology Group. (2003). Randomized, controlled trial of an easy-to-read informed consent statement for clinical trial participation: A study of the Eastern Cooperative Oncology Group. *Journal of Clinical Oncology, 21*(5), 836–842.

Doss, S., DePascal, P., & Hadley, K. (2011). Patient-nurse partnerships. *Nephrology Nursing Journal, 38*(2), 115–125.

Enama, M. E., Hu, Z., Gordon, I., Costner, P., Ledgerwood, J. E., Grady, C., & VRC 306 and 307 Consent Study Teams. (2012). Randomization to standard and concise consent forms: Development of evidence-based consent practices. *Contemporary Clinical Trials, 33*(5), 895–902.

Evelyn, B., Toigo, T., Banks, D., Pohl, D., Gray, K., Robins, B., & Ernat, J. (2001). Participation of racial/ethnic groups in clinical trials and race related labeling: A review of new molecular entities approved 1995-1999. *Journal of the National Medical Association, 93*(12 Suppl.), 18S–24S.

Ford, M. E., Siminoff, L. A., Pickelsimer, E., Mainous, A. G., Smith, D. W., Diaz, V. A., & Tilley, B. C. (2013). Unequal burden of disease, unequal participation in clinical trials: Solutions from African American and Latino Community Members. *Health and Social Work, 38*(1), 29–38.

Guidance for Industry. E6 Good Clinical Practice. (1996). *Consolidated guidance.* Geneva, Switzerland: International Conference on Harmonization of Technical Requirements for Registration of Pharmaceuticals for Human Use.

Hernandez, L. M. (2008). *Standardizing medication labels: Confusing patients less.* Workshop Summary. Washington, DC: The National Academies Press. Retrieved from http://www.nap.edu/catalog/12077.html

Houts, P. S., Doak, C. C., Doak, L. G., & Loscalzo, M. (2006) The role of pictures in improving health communication: A review of research on attention, comprehension, recall and adherence. *Patient Education and Counseling, 61*, 173–190.

Jefford, M., & Moore, R. (2008). Improvement of informed consent and the quality of consent documents. *Lancet Oncology, 9*, 485–493.

Joffe, S., Cook, E. F., Cleary, P. D., Clark, J. W., & Weeks, J. C. (2001). Quality of informed consent: A new measure of understanding among research subjects. *Journal of the National Cancer Institute, 93*(2), 139–147.

Juraskova, I., Butow, P., Lopez, A., Seccombe, M., Coates, A., Boyle, F., . . . Forbes, J. F. (2008). Improving informed consent: Pilot of a decision aid for women invited to participate in a breast cancer prevention trial (IBIS-II DCIS). *Health Expectations, 11*(3), 252–262.

Killien, M., Bigby, J. A., Champion, V., Fernandez-Repollet, E., Jackson, R. D., Kagawa-Singer, M., . . . Prout, M. (2000). Involving minority and underrepresented women in clinical trials: The National Centers of Excellence in Women's Health. *Journal of Women's Health and Gender Based Medicine, 9*(10), 1061–1070.

Koziatek, S., & Young, M. (2012). VOICE offers model for thorough, subject-friendly consent process. *IRB Advisor, 12*(10), 109–112.

National Commission for the Protection of Human Subjects of Biomedical and Behavioral Research. (1979, April). *The Belmont Report: Ethical principles and guidelines for the protection of human subjects of research.* Washington, DC: U.S. Government Printing Office.

Nielsen-Bohlman, L., Panzer, A., & Kindig, D. A. (2004). *Health literacy: A prescription to end confusion.* Washington, DC: The National Academies Press.

Nolte, E., & McKee, C. M. (2008). Measuring the health of nations: Updating an earlier analysis. *Health Affairs (Project Hope), 27*(1), 58–71.

O'Connor, A. M., Rostom, A., Fiset, V., Tetroe, J., Entwistle, V., Llewellyn-Thomas, H., . . . Jones, J. (1999). Decision aids for patients facing health treatment of screening decisions. Systematic Review. *BMJ, 319*(7212), 731–734.

Paasche-Orlow, M. K. (2005). Tailored education may reduce health literacy disparities in asthma self-management. *American Journal of Respiratory and Critical Care Medicine, 172,* 980–986.

Palmer, B. W., Lanouette, N. M., & Jeste, D. V. (2012). Effectiveness of multimedia aids to enhance comprehension of research consent information: A systematic review. *IRB Ethics and Human Research, 34*(6), 1–9.

Ridpath, J. R., Greene, S. M., & Wiese, C. J. (2007). *PRISM readability toolkit* (3rd ed.). Seattle, WA: Group Health Research Institute.

Rowbotham, M. C., Astin, J., Greene, K., & Cummings, S. R. (2013). Interactive informed consent: Randomized comparison with paper consents. *PLoS One, 8*(3), 1–6.

Schenker, Y., & Meisel, A. (2011). Informed consent in clinical care: Practical considerations in the effort to achieve ethical goals. *JAMA, 305*(11), 1130–1131.

Schillinger, D. M., & Keller, D. (2011). *The other side of the coin: Attributes of a health literate healthcare organization.* Washington, DC: The National Academies Press.

Smedly, B. D., Stith, A. Y., & Nelson, A. R. (2003). *Unequal treatment: Confronting racial and ethinic disparities in healthcare.* Washington, DC: The National Academies Press.

Stryker, J. E., Wray, R. J., Emmons, K. M., Winer, E., & Demetri, G. (2006). Understanding the decisions of cancer clinical trial participants to enter research studies: Factors associated with informed consent, patient satisfaction and decisional regret. *Patient Education Counseling, 63,* 104–109.

Sudore, R. L., Landefeld, C. S., Williams, B. A., Barnes, D. E., Lindquist, K., & Schillinger, D. (2006). Use of a modified informed consent process among vulnerable patients. *Journal of General Internal Medicine, 21*(8), 867–873.

U.S. Department of Health and Human Services. 45 Code of Federal Regulations 46 (1991). *Federal Register.* Retrieved from http://www.hhs.gov/ohrp /humansubjects/guidance/45cfr46.html

U.S. Department of Health and Human Services. (2003). *Outreach notebook for the inclusion, recruitment and retention of women and minority research subjects in clinical research* (NIH Publiciation No. 03-70-36). Bethesda, MD: National Institutes of Health.

Wallace, K., Fleshner, N., Jewett, M., Basiuk, J., & Crook, J. (2006). Impact of a multi-disciplinary patient education session on accrual to a difficult clinical trial: The Toronto experience with the Surgical Prostatectomy Versus Interstitial Radiation Intervention Trial. *Journal of Clinical Oncology, 24*(25), 4158–4162.

Wolf, M. S., Davis, T. C., Shrank, W., Rapp, D. N., Bass, P. F., Connor, U. M., . . . Parker, R. M. (2007). To err is human: Patient misinterpretations of prescription drug label instructions. *Patient Education and Counseling, 67,* 293–300.

Index